Homeopathy
H A N D B O O K

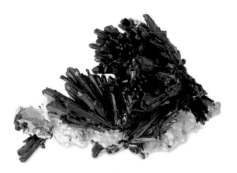

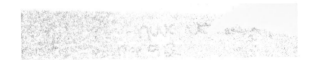

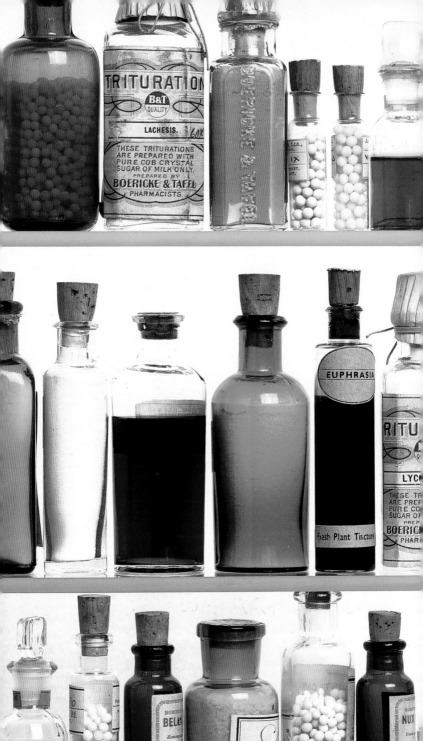

Homeopathy
HANDBOOK

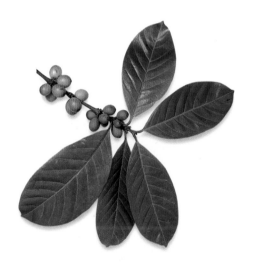

DR. ANDREW LOCKIE

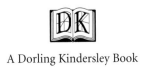

A Dorling Kindersley Book

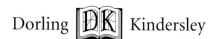

Dorling **DK** Kindersley

LONDON, NEW YORK, SYDNEY, DELHI, PARIS,
MUNICH AND JOHANNESBURG

Produced for Dorling Kindersley by Walton and Pringle
www.waltonandpringle.com

Managing Editor Gillian Roberts
Managing Art Editor Tracey Ward
Category Publisher Mary-Clare Jerram
Art Director Tracy Killick
DTP Designers Louise Paddick and Louise Waller
Production Manager Maryann Webster

First published in Great Britain in 2001 by
Dorling Kindersley Limited,
9 Henrietta Street, London WC2E 8PS

A CIP catalogue record for this book is available from The British Library

ISBN 0 7513 2142 7

Colour reproduced by Colourscan, Singapore
Printed and bound in Italy by Graphicom

see our complete
catalogue at
www.dk.com

Contents

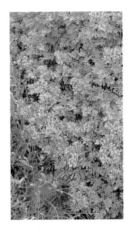
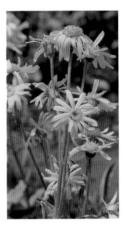

AUTHOR'S INTRODUCTION

An integrated approach to medicine can provide a flexible, pragmatic approach to healthcare; as such homeopathy has an important role to play. By understanding the basics, you will be able to take more responsibility for your own health.

HOMEOPATHY'S ORIGINS

Medical practitioners have long looked to homeopathic-type practices to cure patients. Hippocrates (*see page 12*)and Paracelsus (*see page 10*) made discoveries which continue to affect the practice of homeopathy, but it was not until the late 18th century that a concerted breakthrough was made. It took place in Germany when Dr Samuel Christian Hahnemann (1755–1843), disillusioned with his profession, left his career in conventional medicine to research alternative treatments. He began treating patients with a principle of "like cures like".

In 1796, Hahnemann published his first book about his new type of medicine, *A New Principle for Ascertaining the Curative Powers of Drugs and Some Examinations of Previous Principles*. He called his new system "homeopathy", from the Greek *homeo* meaning "similar" and *pathos* meaning "suffering".

UNDERSTANDING THE BASICS

The key to homeopathy is the practitioner's ability to understand and interpret a patient's symptoms – the outward signs of internal disorder – both before and after a remedy is given. Whereas in conventional medical practice, people diagnosed with the same condition will generally be given the same medicine, in homeopathy the patient is treated holistically. Homeopathic practitioners take into consideration a whole host of other factors, such as temperament, state of mind, and lifestyle, before suggesting a remedy.

Homeopathy's safe, gentle approach complies with one of the most important rules of medical intervention: namely that it should do no harm. A great many common, everyday ailments may be treated safely and effectively at home with homeopathic remedies.

FOR THE LAYPERSON

The author's aim is to provide the layperson with a comprehensive account of homeopathy and its uses. By understanding the basics of the practice you can assist your body's well-being. There are many hundreds of homeopathic remedies available commercially and attempting to choose the correct one can be confusing. This book aims to unravel some of the mysteries surrounding homeopathy and enables the layperson to make a more informed choice about homeopathic self-treatment.

SERIOUS AILMENTS

Under no circumstances, however, should patients suffering from serious ailments (or those uncertain of their ailment) consider self-treatment. They should always consult a recommended homeopathic practitioner or a conventional doctor.

In general a conventional doctor should be consulted for any ailment that can be treated quickly and effectively by conventional medicine or for any condition that requires further investigation. This also applies to common ailments which worsen: a cold that develops into a chest infection, for example.

Certain serious ailments may be alleviated by homeopathy, but in the treatment of these conditions, the experience of a qualified homeopathic practitioner is essential from the outset.

COMPLEMENTARY MEDICINE

It is a truism that no one in the system of medicine can cure every illness every time in every patient. Some patients respond well to certain treatments whereas others, with seemingly similar symptoms, do not. In many parts of the world, conventionally trained doctors are increasingly turning to complementary therapies, such as homeopathy, to widen the range of treatments available to them.

WHY THE CHANGE?

This response by the medical profession is, to some extent, in answer to the desires of a growing number of patients; people who wish to take more responsibility for their own health. An increasing number want to understand what they can do themselves to prevent illness and, if they do become ill, to understand the causes and determine how they can help themselves recover. Homeopathy offers a simple, effective, extremely safe, and relatively inexpensive way of accomplishing this – provided it is practised with common sense.

SCIENTIFIC RESEARCH

The author has carried out much research into the scientific classifications of the substances from which homeopathic remedies are made. This was undertaken in order to correct the various errors and confusions that have crept into homeopathic medicine over the past 200 years. Incorporated into this book is the most up-to-date and scientifically accurate information available – for instance, the current biological, zoological, and mineralogical classifications have been used wherever possible. As a result you may find that some of the Latin names used here are different from those found in earlier homeopathic textbooks.

Understanding
Homeopathy

A guide to the development of homeopathic

treatment, explaining how remedies are made,

how patients are assessed, how to self-assess,

how to take homeopathic remedies, and how

to help remedies work effectively.

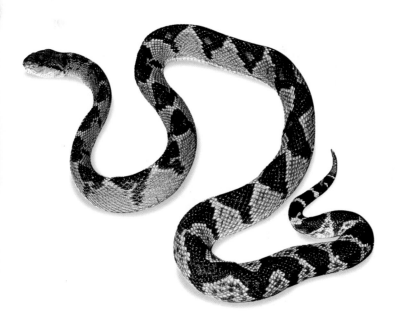

WHAT IS HOMEOPATHY?

Homeopathy is a holistic form of complementary medicine, aiming to treat the whole person, rather than just the physical symptoms. Its theories and principles date back to medicinal practices of ancient Greece and Rome.

IN THE BEGINNING

In the 5th century BC, the Greek physician Hippocrates (469–377 BC) established the idea that disease resulted from natural forces rather than divine intervention, and that the patients' own powers of healing should be encouraged. At the time, medical theories were based upon the Law of Contraries, which advocated treating an illness by prescribing a substance that produced opposite or contrary symptoms to it; in contrast Hippocrates developed the use of the Law of Similars, based on the principle that "like cures like".

PARACELSUS

For many centuries after the decline of the Roman Empire, little progress was made in the field of European medicine. Religion exerted a great influence over medical practice and much early knowledge was forgotten.

It was when Swiss alchemist and physician, Paracelsus (1493–1541), began to develop his theories that the study of medicine started to evolve again. He revived the ancient

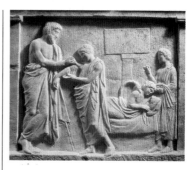

This Greek votive relief (early 4th century BC) illustrates ancient Greek medicinal traditions. Conventional and homeopathic medicine derive from this time.

Greek theory of the Doctrine of Signatures. This was based on the premise that the external appearance of a plant – God's "signature" – indicated the nature of its healing properties. For example, *Chelidonium majus* (greater celandine) was used to treat conditions affecting the liver and gallbladder because the yellow juice of the plant resembled bile.

Paracelsus believed disease was linked to external factors, such as contaminated food and water, rather than to mystical forces. He claimed that medical practice should be based on detailed observation and "profound knowledge of nature and her works". He believed all plants and metals contained active ingredients that could be prescribed to match specific illnesses and maintained "it depends only on the dose whether a poison is a poison or not". According to British homeopath and author James Compton Burnett (1840–1901), "Paracelsus planted the acorn from which the mighty oak of homeopathy has grown".

SAMUEL HAHNEMANN

In Germany of 1780, Dr Samuel Hahnemann began practising homeopathy. For nine years he worked as a conventional doctor, but grew increasingly disillusioned with the harsh medical methods of the day. He maintained that improving public hygiene, housing conditions, general health, and nutrition would do more good than the current medical practices alone.

In 1790, Hahnemann began researching a new type of medicine he called "homeopathy". He conducted tests ("provings") on himself and, later, on patients. Prior to prescription, he gave his patients a thorough physical examination and noted any existing symptoms. He questioned them closely regarding their lifestyles, general health, outlook on life, and other factors that made them feel better or worse. Following the principle of "like cures like", Hahnemann matched individual symptoms as closely as possible to the symptom picture of a particular remedy and prescribed accordingly.

HAHNEMANN'S REMEDIES

In 1812 Hahnemann began teaching homeopathy at the University of Leipzig. During the course of his lifetime he proved about 100 remedies. He also continued to develop and refine the theory and practice of the system. Despite this, the established medical world remained generally very sceptical of Hahnemann; in turn he remained equally scornful of the established medical world.

HOMEOPATHY TODAY

By the time of Hahnemann's death (1843) homeopathy was firmly established in many parts of the world. There have been occasional periods of disenchantment but, generally, its popularity continues to spread and recent trends show a strong resurgence, particularly in the US. Single-remedy prescribing is prevalent worldwide, although in Germany and France the use of complex homeopathy, also known as polypharmacy (the use of combination or several remedies), is also popular. In Australia homeopathy has become strongly linked with naturopathy; whilst in India homeopaths have long worked successfully alongside traditional Ayurvedic medicine and conventional medicine. In the 1990s, pioneering British teachers revitalized an interest in homeopathy in Eastern Europe; in Russia it continues to be developed. In South America homeopathy has become so popular that it is taught widely in medical schools.

HOW DOES IT WORK?

Homeopaths believe that good health derives from an equilibrium between the mind and body, which is maintained by a "vital force" that regulates the body's self-healing capabilities.

THE VITALISTIC CONCEPT

The vitalistic concept of science had already existed for many years by Hahnemann's time. It claims that all living things possess a subtle energy beyond their physical and chemical states, and that even inanimate matter may contain vitality. Hahnemann applied this view to both the human body and to seemingly inert substances from all the kingdoms of matter. Thus the vital force of any plant, mineral, or animal could be harnessed to produce a powerful medicine when "potentized".

Hahnemann viewed ill-health as the result of an internal imbalance affecting the body's vital force and disrupting its equilibrium. He believed that if this vital force is put under strain or weakened by this imbalance, illness may develop. In stimulating the body's self-healing abilities to fight any imbalance, Hahnemann proclaimed that the vital force produces symptoms. These may manifest themselves externally, producing such symptoms as fever or a skin rash, or may emerge as emotional or psychological states, such as weepiness or great irritability. An effective medicine must help the vital force to redress the internal imbalance, enabling the symptoms produced by that imbalance to disappear; this is what homeopaths seek to achieve.

A PERSON'S CONSTITUTION

Homeopathy works on the principle that the mind and body are so strongly linked that physical symptoms cannot be sucessfully treated without an understanding of the person's constitution and

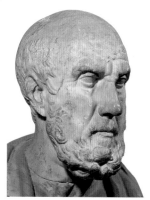

Portrait bust of Hippocrates (460–377 BC), known as the "father of medicine". He established the foundations of conventional and homeopathic medicine.

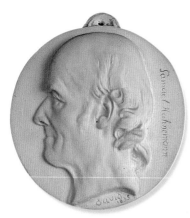

Portrait medallion of Dr Samuel Christian Hahnemann (1755–1843). Disenchanted with conventional medicine, he began work on a new system he called "homeopathy".

character. In homeopathic terms, a person's "constitution" describes their state of health, including their temperament and any inherited and acquired characteristics. In determining constitution, a practitioner needs to ask a great many questions (*see pages 18–19*).

Homeopaths believe that healthy people resist developing sickness – despite being constantly exposed to an enormous variety of potentially harmful viruses and bacteria – as their vital force is strong and their susceptibility is therefore low.

LIKE CURES LIKE

Hahnemann developed the concept of "like cures like" (*similia similibus curentur*), first established by Hippocrates. According to this theory, substances that are capable of provoking certain symptoms in an otherwise healthy body can also act curatively on similar symptoms in a sick person. For example, *Belladonna* would be used to treat

scarlet fever, since the symptoms of *Belladonna* poisoning closely resemble those of scarlet fever.

SYMPTOM PICTURES

Hahnemann's "provings" of remedies aimed to establish the particular set of symptoms – known as a "symptom picture" – produced by taking a particular substance. When the symptom picture matched the particular set of symptoms produced by an illness or imbalance in a patient, that remedy was indicated as the most effective at stimulating the vital force to treat the disorder. The key of classical homeopathy is to establish which remedy most exactly matches a patient's symptom picture.

LAWS OF CURE

As a patient progresses towards being completely cured, symptoms move from the body's inner organs (most vital) to the outer organs (less vital). Cure usually takes place from the top of the body to the bottom; as an example, head symptoms clear first, these are followed gradually by any symptoms on the extremities.

Old symptoms of illness often resurface during the homeopathic curative process, usually in the reverse order to that in which they first appeared. Immunologists claim that the body has the capacity to "remember" every "assault" on the system that it has reacted to – this process of symptoms resurfacing confirms this theory.

13

HOW REMEDIES ARE MADE

Homeopathic remedies are prepared to exact guidelines, but may vary in strength according to individual needs. A practitioner's skill, experience, and judgment in selecting the appropriate remedy are of paramount importance.

HAHNEMANN'S METHOD

Many of the substances from which remedies are made are highly poisonous. Hahnemann used only small amounts in his medicines, but to his consternation his patients still tended to suffer side-effects, or "aggravations" as he called them. He developed a technique called "potentization", which involved diluting the medicine and shaking it vigorously or banging it on a hard surface during preparation. This turbulent motion, which Hahnemann called "succussion" (*see below*), apparently released more potency into the medicine, even at lower dilutions, allowing a lower dosage to be administered.

PREPARING MATERIALS

Some plant materials may be used whole in the creation of remedies, but most raw animal and plant materials (such as leaves, roots, and flower heads) require chopping as preparation. Crystalline minerals, as well as beans or seeds, may require grinding if they are large, hard, or insoluble in water.

HOW TO MAKE TABLETS FROM ALLIUMS

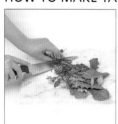

1 PREPARE RAW MATERIAL

Plant materials or animal matter must be chopped finely. Other substances can be prepared by being dissolved in water or by being ground.

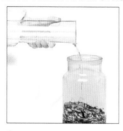

2 MIX WITH ALCOHOL

Mix the substance with alcohol and distilled water (ratios vary but 90 per cent alcohol to 10 per cent water is common). Use a large glass container for mixing.

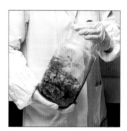

3 LEAVE TO STAND

Plant materials may stand for several weeks; mineral-based mixtures may be processed almost immediately. Longer-standing mixtures should be shaken periodically.

TRITURATION

This term describes the process of changing insoluble metals into powder. Metals that are insoluble in their natural states are combined with lactose sugar crystals; they are then ground repeatedly until they form a powder that is fine enough to be soluble in water.

COMBINING INGREDIENTS

When the raw ingredients have been prepared, they are mixed with a solution of alcohol and distilled water. The ratio of this solution varies according to the substance with which it is being mixed. The mixture is then left to stand for anything from a few moments to several weeks. This stage is known as "maceration". Mineral-based mixtures may be moved on to the next stage almost at once, whereas certain plant-based mixtures may need weeks. Those that are left to stand for a while may require occasional shaking.

THE MOTHER TINCTURE

Liquid is extracted from the mixture (either by straining or pressing) to produce what is known as the "mother tincture". This is then added to a second solution of pure alcohol and distilled water, made up according to one of several scales. The most commonly used are the decimal scale (in which the dilution factor is 1:10) and the centesimal scale (in which the dilution factor is 1:100). The tincture is succussed and diluted as many times as is necessary to achieve the required potency for the homeopathic remedy.

EXERCISE CAUTION

This information is not intended as a guide to making remedies. Unlike herbal remedies, homeopathic remedies should never be made in the home; they are prepared under strict conditions by a commercial manufacturer and should be obtained from a reputable supplier.

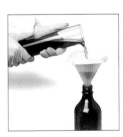

4 STRAIN THE LIQUID

When it is ready, strain the mixture through a filter or push it through a press to extract the liquid. This is the "mother tincture"; it should be stored in a dark glass jar.

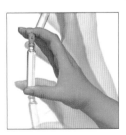

5 SUCCUSS THE MIXTURE

To succuss the liquid, shake it vigorously or bang the jar firmly on a hard surface. Hahnemann coined the term "succussion"; he believed it "potentized" the liquid.

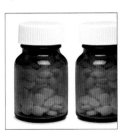

6 IMPREGNATE TABLETS

When the tincture is the correct strength and potency, add the required amount of drops to lactose tablets, pilules, granules, or powder. Store in dark glass bottles.

REMEDY STRENGTHS

Remedies are prepared to exact guidelines, but vary in strength according to the patient's needs. The practitioner's skill, experience, and judgement are responsible for selecting the appropriate remedy and its strength.

HAHNEMANN'S RULES

Hahnemann wrote precise guidelines in which methods and measurements were all strictly and scientifically controlled. He developed a unique process called "potentization", which allowed the full strength, or potency, of the substance to be released into the remedy mixture.

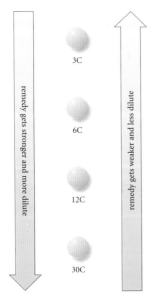

The more dilute a remedy, the stronger it is, and the higher the number or "potency"; a less dilute remedy is not as strong and has a lower number ("potency").

DILUTION

As many remedies are based on extremely poisonous or highly active ingredients, they needed to be diluted to eliminate the risk of patients suffering adverse effects. Because they are diluted to such a great degree, it is highly unlikely that even a single molecule of the original substance remains. This means that, although remedies may be based on highly poisonous substances, they are completely safe to use, even on children.

THE NUMBERING SYSTEM

Hahnemann made a surprising discovery: the more dilute the remedy, the fewer doses are needed. More dilute remedies are therefore stronger, producing a longer action and deeper effect than less dilute remedies. When recording his works, Hahnemann gave stronger remedies high numbers, denoting their higher potency, and vice versa.

Remedies usually have a number, such as *6c* or *12x*, after the name. This number indicates how many times a remedy has been diluted and succussed, and on which scale

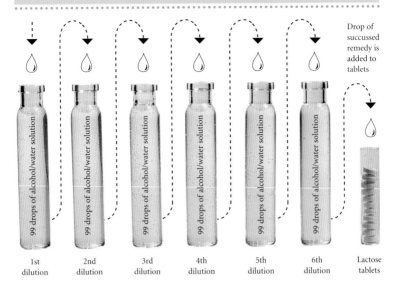

| 1st dilution | 2nd dilution | 3rd dilution | 4th dilution | 5th dilution | 6th dilution | Lactose tablets |

Drop of succussed remedy is added to tablets

(see above). For example, the remedy *Allium cepa 6c* has been diluted and succussed six times on the centesimal scale.

SCALES OF DILUTION

Homeopathic remedies are generally prepared according to one of two scales: the decimal (*x*) and the centesimal (*c*) (*see page 15*). More rarely, however, scales such as the millesimal (*m*) and quinquagintamillesimal (*lm*) are prepared. According to these scales, remedies are diluted by factors of 1:1,000 and 1:50,000 respectively. The millesimal is advocated mainly when a single, high-potency dose of a remedy is required; the quinquagintamillesimal is used for stubborn, chronic cases that seem to require the prescription of a "megadose" of a particular remedy.

PREPARING A POTENCY

The mother tincture (*see page 15*) is usually diluted in a mixture (the

The mother tincture is usually diluted with a mixture of alcohol and water; it is then succussed. This is repeated as many times as necessary to produce the required potency.

ratio of which varies) made from pure alcohol and distilled water, according to one of the scales. To produce a 1c potency, one drop of the mother tincture is added to 99 drops of an alcohol-and-water mixture and succussed. To produce a 2c potency, one drop of the 1c mixture is added to 99 drops of alcohol and water and succussed. This is repeated until the required potency results.

CHOOSING THE POTENCY

The potency prescribed is gauged by the homeopath according to several factors, such as the condition to be treated, the strength of the patient, and the circumstances. Not only must the remedy given be suitable, but the potency chosen must also be appropriate to the individual patient.

HOW PATIENTS ARE ASSESSED

As the basis of homeopathic assessment, a practitioner collects a wealth of information about a patient, to build up an overview of the symptoms. The charts below show the type of information a homeopath will require.

BODY

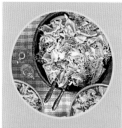

Diet plays an important role in physical well-being

PHYSICAL WELL-BEING
- General symptoms and ailments.
- Weight, shape, and physical condition.
- Diet: food preferences and aversions, food intolerances, deficiencies, any special requirements.
- Energy levels.
- Sleep: amount, quality, dreams.
- Risks to health: smoking, alcohol consumption, recreational drugs, dangerous jobs and pastimes.
- Time out: relaxation methods, leisure activities.
- Knowledge of what to do if ill or injured.

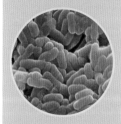

A homeopath needs to know your medical history

MEDICAL HISTORY
- Personal medical history and history of treatments.
- Family medical history: incidence in family of conditions such as heart disease, diabetes, mental health problems, or cancer.
- Inherited susceptibilities, such as allergies.
- Diet: food intolerances, susceptibility to obesity.
- Awareness of symptoms of genetically inherited disease and preventative measures.
- Check-ups: self-examination, regular medical tests or screening.

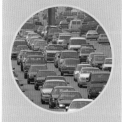

Knowing about a patient's environment is vital

ENVIRONMENT
- Climate: effects of seasonal changes and day-to-day weather patterns.
- Access to and appreciation of fresh air.
- Exposure to sun and awareness of risks.
- Effects of pollution: air, water, noise.
- Work environment: location, amount of space.
- Home environment: allergies to household products, toiletries, animals, tobacco smoke.
- Daily routine: stress and other effects of commuting, working long hours.

THE INDIVIDUAL PATIENT

◆ **THE PERSON AS PRODUCT**
Homeopaths regard a person as the product of their physical and mental well-being or ill-health, genetic experience, and daily experience.

◆ **PROFILING PATIENTS**
A person's symptoms are seen as reliable clues to the most suitable remedy to activate the self-healing powers of the individual's "vital force". Characteristics of bodily functions and functional disturbances are also noted.

ADAPTATIONS

An individual's unique adaptations to their surroundings and their idiosyncratic ways are accepted and respected for making an individual what they are. The way they adapt to new home, family, or work environments; their reactions to external circumstances; their past and present experiences; and their general state of mind are all key attributes of patient assessment.

MIND

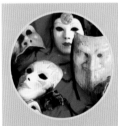

Everyone responds to events in different ways

PERSONALITY
◆ Temperament: relaxed, nervous, passive, assertive.
◆ Self-image and self-worth.
◆ Emotions: positive, negative, expression of, control.
◆ Relationships: sex drive, ability to resolve conflict, sensitivity to others, desire for approval.
◆ Fears, any feelings of guilt, insecurity, degree of control over personal destiny.
◆ Ability to cope under stress.
◆ Opportunities for personal expression.
◆ Spirituality, deeply held beliefs, motivation.

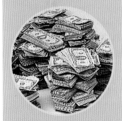

Events that happen early in life can have later effects

LIFE EVENTS
◆ Childhood trauma: death or other loss, abuse.
◆ Family circumstances: births, marriages, separations, divorce, death, bullying, exams, children leaving home, caring for elderly or disabled relatives.
◆ Proximity of family and friends.
◆ Ability to deal with serious health problems.
◆ Property: buying, moving, serious alterations.
◆ Work experience: new job, loss of job, redundancy, relocation, overwork, juggling work and family.
◆ Financial or legal problems.

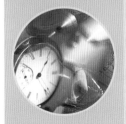

These points are crucial to creating symptom pictures

LIFE MANAGEMENT
◆ Time management, ability to: set realistic goals, plan and organize, cope with deadlines, delegate tasks.
◆ Ability to maintain a successful balance: between work and play, work and family.
◆ Stress management: opportunities to relax, control of stressful situations, turning problems around.
◆ Work: environment, physical stresses, workload.
◆ Routines that have been developed in order to give structure to the working day and home.
◆ Financial planning and organization.

HOW TO SELF-ASSESS

Homeopathic remedies can be used effectively and safely by lay people to treat many minor ailments and injuries. Careful observation enables a person to select a remedy to match their own symptoms.

SELF-PRESCRIPTION

Before starting homeopathic treatment, you must first decide whether or not it is safe to self-prescribe. Some symptoms may be indicative of a serious ailment and require the immediate attention of a conventional doctor. If pharmaceutical drugs are already being taken, it may be necessary to consult a doctor before considering extra medication. Babies, small children, pregnant women, the elderly, and those with chronic medical conditions need extra careful consideration.

IDENTIFYING SYMPTOMS

A diagnostic picture needs to be compiled in order to self-prescribe. A homeopathic practitioner would ask a person to describe themselves in terms of basic temperament, moods, feelings, and beliefs. This includes temporary psychological factors associated with their symptoms, such as irritability or an aversion to sympathy. Also of significance are details about any emotional traumas – from deep-seated, childhood experiences to

events of the recent past, such as bereavement. Details of how the weather, seasons, and times of day affect the individual, personal likes and dislikes, and in particular objects of fear, are all important in building up a complex picture.

ASSESSING LIFESTYLE

When assessing yourself, general features of your lifestyle should be taken into consideration. Dietary factors of significance include caffeine, alcohol, and tobacco consumption, food preferences and aversions, and potential sources of irritation or digestive upset. Stress levels are also significant. You should look carefully at the amount of stress caused by work, at the time you have for relaxation and for following interests, whether you get enough sleep, and the amount, and type, of exercise you take.

SYMPTOM PICTURES

A "symptom picture" is compiled from all the information provided by a patient, making use of external information as well as the bodily ailments. Make a note of the characteristics of the symptoms suffered or noticed (if prescribing for someone else, also make a note of what you can see and everything they tell you). Some symptoms may be associated with other ailments or with a particular state of mind and it is necessary to ascertain all such information before deciding on a course of action. Armed with a symptom picture, a person can look at the charts and remedies profiled in this book, and identify suitable treatment. It should be noted that it is not necessary to exhibit all the symptoms listed in order for a particular remedy to be suitable. One can be chosen on the basis of the main symptoms, the likely cause, and the onset characteristics.

SAFETY ISSUES

There are several rules to remember before self-prescribing.

• Consult a conventional doctor for serious or unknown ailments, or if there is no improvement in two to three weeks (48 hours in children under five).

• Do not use aromatherapy or herbal products during the first three months of pregnancy, or when trying to conceive.

• Do not exceed the recommended dosage of any remedy without seeking professional supervision.

• Do not stop taking any prescribed conventional medicine without first consulting a conventional doctor.

• Tell your doctor about any homeopathic remedies you take.

DIAGNOSTIC CHECKLIST

QUESTIONS	EXAMPLE ANSWERS
WHAT ARE YOUR MOST OBVIOUS PHYSICAL SYMPTOMS?	Pain, soreness, inflammation, skin eruption, itching, bleeding, nausea, vomiting, diarrhoea, sore throat, cough, fever, fainting, dizziness, headache.
ARE MAIN SYMPTOMS ACCOMPANIED BY LESS ACUTE SYMPTOMS?	Perspiration, chilliness, great thirst, desire for or aversion to certain foods, loss of appetite, sensitivity to touch, weak limbs, coated tongue, swollen glands.
WHAT ARE THE CHAR-ACTERISTICS OF YOUR SYMPTOMS?	Location in the body, sudden or gradual onset, constant or intermittent occurrence, frequency or recurrence.
DO YOU HAVE ANY PSYCHOLOGICAL SYMPTOMS?	Restlessness, irritability, anger, anxiety, tearfulness, self-pity, emotional oversensitivity, indifference, desire to be alone, irrational fears, desire for sympathy.
ARE YOU AWARE OF ANY OBVIOUS CAUSE OF YOUR SYMPTOMS?	Injury, viral infection, bacterial infection, exposure to extremes of temperature or strong wind, stress, anxiety, grief, overwork.
DO YOUR SYMPTOMS IMPROVE OR WORSEN IN CERTAIN CONDITIONS?	Warmth or cold, fresh air, application of hot or cold compresses, sitting or standing, lying in a particular way, physical or mental exertion, emotional stress.

HOW TO TAKE REMEDIES

Homeopathic remedies come in several different forms; the choice of which type to use depends upon personal preference as well as upon the patient's aptitude for taking medication.

TYPES OF REMEDIES

Lactose tablets are the most common form of homeopathic remedy, although sucrose tablets are available for those who suffer from lactose-intolerance. Because these tablets can be dissolved under the tongue, a remedy is able to enter the bloodstream directly.

Remedies are also available as pilules, granules, or powder, and mother tinctures may be diluted to make soothing solutions, or used in the creation of ointments and creams. The latter can be applied directly onto the skin. You may also see remedies sold as "biochemic tissue salts", these are minerals that can be taken on their own or as part of a combination with other homeopathic remedies to treat common ailments.

INDIVIDUAL NEEDS

Given the highly individualistic nature of homeopathic prescription, two people are unlikely to be prescribed the same remedy, even if their symptoms appear to be identical. For the same reason, patients may find that their

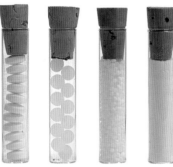

Different forms of homeopathic remedy, shown from left to right: tablets, pilules, granules, and powder.

remedies do not match any of the general profiles of remedies listed for their ailment in popular homeopathic course books.

One remedy may be prescribed constitutionally to address the underlying causes of an ailment, for instance bodily imbalances, with another remedy prescribed for a specific, acute symptom. Also, one remedy may be substituted for another on a subsequent visit to the practitioner, depending on the patient's progress.

PROMOTING RECOVERY

Unless a qualified practitioner has recommended a combination of homeopathic remedies (*see above*) it is best to take only one at a time. One reason for this is that a remedy's effectiveness may be lessened if used in combination. Taking remedies individually also allows for assessment of the efficacy of the remedy: the decision to repeat the dosage (or the remedy itself) relies on the practitioner being able to discover whether or not a remedy has worked by working out whether the symptoms have improved.

All homeopathic remedies work best when combined with good nutrition, exercise, a low-stress environment, and emotional and intellectual states that promote a balanced body system.

FOLLOWING THE RULES

In order to take homeopathic remedies effectively, it is important to follow the rules for maximizing effects (*see tint panel*). The reasons for doing so are are as follows:
• Patients should leave at least 30 minutes after eating before taking a remedy so that it enters the system on its own.
• Likewise it is important not to eat for 30 minutes after taking a remedy so as not to inhibit absorbtion.
• The recommendation to avoid strong foods and drinks is due to the fact that they may affect the body's system – some, such as coffee, may actually counteract the remedy.
• Strong household cleaners and other such chemical products may actually have a poisoning effect on the body.
• Avoiding certain medical substances is important because these may inhibit a remedy from working on its own. If in doubt, consult your practitioner.
• Avoid touching homeopathic remedies as this can prevent them from working effectively. Remedies should be taken with a clean, dry spoon, or dropped into the mouth, without being touched by the fingers. If tablets are touched or dropped, they should not be returned to the container.
• When storing homeopathic remedies, make sure that the tops are securely in place. Also ensure that they are kept in a suitable location and temperature.

MAXIMIZING EFFECTS

When taking a homeopathic remedy, observe the following "rules" in order to ensure that it has the best chance of working effectively.

• Do not eat for 30 mins before taking a remedy.

• Do not eat for 30 mins after taking a remedy.

• Avoid strong foods and drinks, such as spicy foods and alcohol or consume them only in moderation.

• Avoid brushing your teeth 30 mins before or after taking a remedy.

• Avoid using strong substances, such as household cleaning products.

• Avoid medicinal substances and certain products such as some essential oils.

• Do not touch or handle a remedy.

• Store homeopathic products properly.

HELPING REMEDIES TO WORK

A homeopathic remedy helps the body to heal itself.
This self-healing can be encouraged, and future health
and well-being promoted, by a series of measures put
into place alongside the treatment.

COMPLEMENTARY LIFESTYLE GUIDE

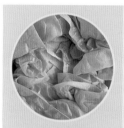

Eating regular meals is important for good health

EATING FOR HEALTH
- Eat vegetarian proteins rather than meat and dairy.
- Eat foods rich in minerals and vitamins, or take supplements.
- Cut down on refined carbohydrates, salt, processed foods, sugar, animal fats, yeast, caffeine, and alcohol.
- Drink plenty of fluids.
- Lose weight if necessary.
- Consult a dietician about specific needs.
- Include plenty of fibre in the diet.
- Cook healthily: for instance, grill instead of frying.

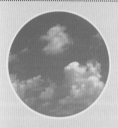

Strong household products are potential irritants

IMPROVING SURROUNDINGS
- Prohibit smoking at home and at work.
- Reduce allergies by keeping the home dust free.
- Use environmentally friendly household products.
- Avoid perfumed toiletries and skin-care products.
- Avoid polluted or noisy environments.
- Humidify or de-humidify rooms as necessary.
- Make sure rooms are draught-free but have adequate ventilation.
- Wear natural fibres.
- Create an area that is conducive to relaxation.

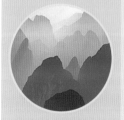

Seeing close family and friends helps relieve stress

MANAGING STRESS
- Take periods of rest during the day and get enough sleep at night.
- Make time for relaxation and exercise each day.
- Prioritize and organize tasks.
- Delegate and learn to say "no" to extra work.
- Eat properly and regularly; get plenty of fresh air.
- Make time for leisure activities and socializing.
- Take a holiday.
- Cultivate a positive attitude to all things.
- Face up to problems rather than putting them off.

PROMOTING GOOD HEALTH

◆ SELF-HEALING

While not necessarily providing a instant cure, a homeopathic remedy is believed to encourage the body's self-healing mechanisms and to nurture a sense of well-being, good energy levels, and a resistance to ill-health.

◆ A SENSE OF WELL-BEING

In order to heal physical symptoms, it is important to take a look at the mind. A positive mental attitude is a crucial tool in getting better physically.

THE HOLISTIC VIEW

All homeopathic remedies can be helped to work by adopting a lifestyle that will promote good health and a positive outlook. Eating a balanced diet and taking regular exercise are of obvious benefit; however homeopaths also need to look at other aspects of a person's life – such as their outlook on life and external circumstances – before deciding on treatment.

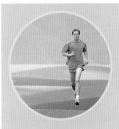

Warm up and cool down before and after exercise

KEEPING FIT

- Learn breathing techniques to maximize the benefits of exercise.
- Include exercise in a daily routine.
- Plan a weekly exercise programme.
- Aim to improve your energy levels, brain-power, and mood.
- Choose activities for specific purposes, such as muscle coordination, strength, or endurance.
- Use exercise as a means of getting time to yourself, or meeting people, or as a challenge.

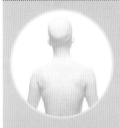

Manipulation can ease spine and joint disorders

TREATMENTS FOR THE BODY

- Breathing and relaxation techniques: for relief of pain and stress-related symptoms.
- Touch therapies: pressure or massage for general wellbeing and health (aromatherapy, reflexology).
- Manipulation: for bone and muscle disorders, and body alignment (physiotherapy, osteopathy).
- Physical re-education: for tension release, posture, and flexibility (Pilates, Alexander technique).
- Movement therapies: for increased vitality and self-healing (t'ai chi, yoga, dance movement therapy).

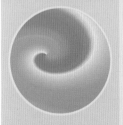

Hypnotherapy can be used to desensitize pain

TREATMENTS FOR THE MIND

- Breathing and relaxation techniques: for managing stress and treating mental conditions.
- Meditation: focusing on feelings of inner peace and fulfilment rather than on thought processes.
- Psychotherapy and counselling: talking to a skilled listener treats mental and emotional disorders.
- Hypnotherapy: using a trance-like, conscious state to influence physical and mental conditions.
- Creative therapies: use of sounds, music, or art to treat mental and emotional disorders.

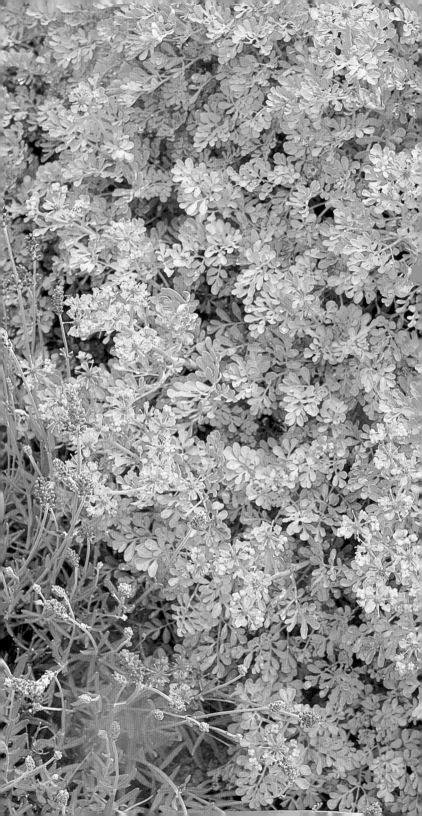

Choosing
a Remedy

A visual guide to 72 key homeopathic remedies

with details of their actions and current uses.

Also included are key homeopathic preparations

and practical self-help advice.

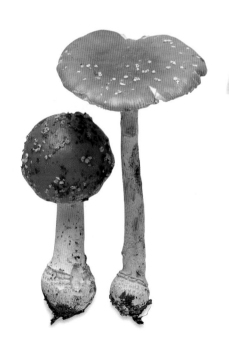

ARSEN. ALB.

Key remedy for asthma and breathlessness

Calms digestive disorders ◆ Treats skin complaints

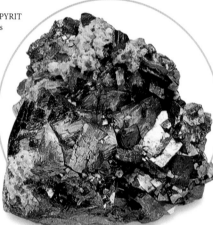

ARSENOPYRITE forms as prismatic crystals.

Crystals have a metallic lustre and when heated or struck, they give off a smell of garlic.

This mineral is the main ore of arsenic.

Arsenopyrite is found in Sweden, Germany, Norway, England, and Canada.

KEY ACTIONS

- AIDS WITH BREATHING
- TREATS VOMITING AND DIARRHOEA
- EASES HEADACHES
- HEALS SKIN PROBLEMS

KEY PREPARATIONS

- TINCTURE Arsenic is triturated by being ground repeatedly with lactose sugar until it is soluble in water. It is then diluted and succussed.

INDICATIONS

● **RESPIRATORY ILLNESS**
Arsen. alb. is a key remedy used for asthma and breathlessness. It is given chiefly to treat disorders of the mucous membranes of the respiratory and digestive tracts.

● **DIGESTIVE DISORDERS**
It is prescribed for violent digestive upsets with diarrhoea and vomiting, such as gastroenteritis and colitis. These are often aggravated by stress and anxiety and may be accompanied by fever.

● **CANDIDIASIS**
Arsen. alb. is prescribed for the treatment of

Candidiasis (or 'thrush'), which is characterized by a burning offensive-smelling discharge and inflammation of the genitals.

● **HEADACHES**
Arsen. alb. is used for easing the pain of headaches and associated dizziness, vomiting, and nausea.

● **ANXIETY**
Effective for treating physical and mental anxiety.

● **CAUTION**
In the past doctors of conventional medicine used arsenic to treat eczema, but it is now considered too toxic.

NITRIC AC.

Calms painful skin ailments ◆ Eases catarrh

Used to treat warts, haemorrhoids, and anal fissures

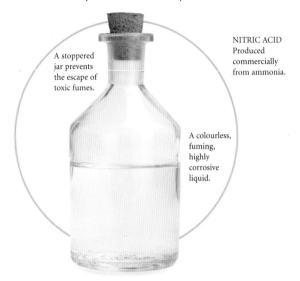

A stoppered jar prevents the escape of toxic fumes.

NITRIC ACID Produced commercially from ammonia.

A colourless, fuming, highly corrosive liquid.

KEY ACTIONS

- RELIEVES CATARRH
- TREATS MOUTH ULCERS
- HELPS RELIEVE HAEMORRHOIDS AND ANAL FISSURES
- HELPS CURE WARTS

KEY PREPARATIONS

- TINCTURE made by diluting one part nitric acid in nine parts alcohol. This mixture is then diluted and succussed.

INDICATIONS

● **CANCER**
Nitric acid is associated with treatment for cancer of the breast, stomach, uterus, and glands in the later stages.

● **SKIN AILMENTS**
Painful skin ailments, especially where the mucous membranes meet the skin of the mouth, nose, or anus, are treated with *Nitric acid*. It is also used to treat warts, anal fissures, haemorrhoids, and mouth ulcers.

● **CATARRH**
Catarrh is characterized by pain in the nostrils and possible nosebleeds. It is worsened by cold, damp air, and the consumption of fatty foods and milk. *Nitric acid* is used to alleviate the symptoms.

● **CANDIDIASIS**
Candidiasis affects males and females. It is a fungus that lives in warm, moist conditions, thriving if the immune system is low. *Nitric acid* is used to treat candidiasis as well as blisters and ulcers on the genitals.

● **CAUTION**
Nitric acid is produced from ammonia, this acid is highly corrosive and gives off fumes that are extremely irritant and toxic if inhaled. The acid should be kept in a stoppered jar.

PHOSPHORIC AC.

Calms exam nerves ◆ Assists conventional medicine

used by diabetics ◆ Relieves headaches

PHOSPHORIC ACID
Used widely in the
drinks industry to give
soft drinks a fruity,
acidic flavour.

Phosphoric acid
is dissolved in
alcohol to make
the remedy.

TRANSPARENT
CRYSTALLINE
SOLID

KEY ACTIONS

- ALLEVIATES INSOMNIA
- RELIEVES MILD DIARRHOEA
- EASES GROWING PAINS
- TREATS EXHAUSTION

KEY PREPARATIONS

- TINCTURE *Phosphoric acid* is dissolved in alcohol in a ratio of 1:9. It is then repeatedly diluted and successed.

INDICATIONS

● **GRIEF**
Phosphoric acid is used in the treatment of grief associated with great exhaustion.

● **DIABETES**
Homeopathic treatment for diabetes is recommended in support of conventional medicine. Prescription depends upon the symptoms, but *Phosphoric acid* is effective when emotional stress has played a part in the onset of diabetes.

● **CFS**
Phosphoric acid is prescribed for weakness in the spinal cord and associated nerves, often symptoms of Chronic Fatigue Syndrome (CFS). The condition is also known as ME (myalgic encephalomyelitis), post-viral syndrome, or yuppie flu.

● **MILD DIARRHOEA**
Travellers should consider taking *Phosphoric acid* in their first aid kit, as it is effective in treating mild cases of diarrhoea.

● **CAUTION**
Homeopathic medicine can assist with grieving. Treatment of long-term depression, however, may require psychiatric help, in conjunction with antidepressant drugs, psychotherapy, and counselling.

ACONITE

Eases childhood sleeplessness ◆ Soothes sore throats and dry, irritating coughs ◆ Helps with emotional problems

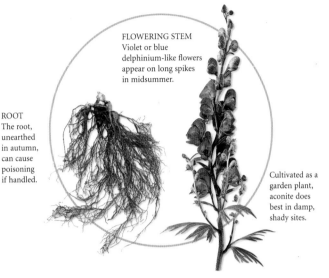

FLOWERING STEM
Violet or blue
delphinium-like flowers
appear on long spikes
in midsummer.

ROOT
The root,
unearthed
in autumn,
can cause
poisoning
if handled.

Cultivated as a
garden plant,
aconite does
best in damp,
shady sites.

KEY ACTIONS

- SOOTHING
- EMOTIONALLY CALMING
- EASES DIFFICULT RESPIRATION
- RELIEVES HEADACHES

KEY PREPARATIONS

- TINCTURE which is made by the whole plant being unearthed during the flowering season, chopped, and macerated in alcohol.

INDICATIONS

● **FEVER**
A sudden rise in temperature, particularly when accompanied by an inflamed throat or a dry, irritating cough, can be alleviated by *Aconite*. Dosage varies according to the symptoms.

● **BRONCHITIS**
Aconite is prescribed to treat bronchitis that comes on suddenly after exposure to cold, dry air.

● **CHILDBIRTH**
Used to relieve a strong fear of impending death experienced by a mother during labour. Also treats urine retention in either the mother or baby.

● **SLEEPLESSNESS**
Poor sleeping patterns in infants or children can be caused by a variety of factors. *Aconite* can help calm a child worried by their inability to sleep or frightened by nightmares.

● **PHOBIAS AND FEARS**
Aconite is used to treat several anxiety states. Particularly for patients who have a fear of dying.

● **HEADACHES**
Pulsating headaches that come on suddenly can be relieved by *Aconite*.

● **CAUTION**
High doses of *Aconite* should not be taken internally due to its toxic nature.

AGARICUS

Used to treat palpitations ◆ Assists alongside conventional medicine for Multiple Sclerosis ◆ Calms anxiety

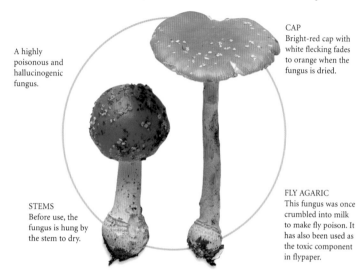

A highly poisonous and hallucinogenic fungus.

CAP
Bright-red cap with white flecking fades to orange when the fungus is dried.

STEMS
Before use, the fungus is hung by the stem to dry.

FLY AGARIC
This fungus was once crumbled into milk to make fly poison. It has also been used as the toxic component in flypaper.

KEY ACTIONS

- USED TO ASSIST SUFFERERS OF PARKINSON'S DISEASE
- CALMING
- ASSISTS WITH HEART IRREGULARITIES
- SOOTHES CHILBLAINS

KEY PREPARATIONS

- TINCTURE made from the Fly Agaric toadstool. The whole, fresh fungus may be used, or the dried cap. It is washed thoroughly and ground into a mash before being steeped in alcohol. It is then strained, diluted, and succussed.

INDICATIONS

● **MUSCLE SPASMS**
These can be indicative of Parkinson's Disease (characterized by general weakness and trembling limbs among other symptoms) or Multiple Sclerosis (characterized by weak, shaky movements accompanied by shooting pains). *Agaricus* may be prescribed to assist conventional medicine.

● **PALPITATIONS**
Palpitations occur for many reasons; *Agaricus* is associated with those induced by stimulants.

● **CHILBLAINS**
Chilblains are common on the hands and feet.

They can be treated effectively with *Agaricus*.

● **TWITCHING EYELIDS**
Agaricus is prescribed for eyelid twitching when there is no other bodily twitching; indicating tiredness or anxiety.

● **CAUTION**
The Fly Agaric toadstool, from which *Agaricus* derives, has been used for centuries in traditional and shamanic medicine. However, it is highly toxic if taken without preparation. A severe overdose can be fatal, while a mild overdose can cause nausea, vomiting, diarrhoea, breathing problems, and confusion.

ALLIUM CEPA

Eases neuralgia ◆ Treats colds and influenza

Alleviates allergies, including hay fever

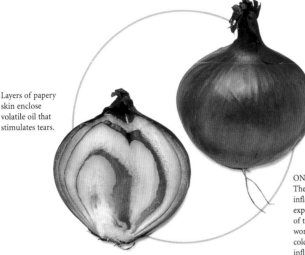

Layers of papery skin enclose volatile oil that stimulates tears.

ONION
The antibiotic, anti-inflammatory, and expectorant properties of this plant are used worldwide to treat colds, coughs, and influenza.

KEY ACTIONS

- EASES CATARRH
- FIGHTS INFECTION
- SOOTHES IRRITATED EYES

KEY PREPARATIONS

- TINCTURE made from the mature bulb, gathered in summer. It is steeped in alcohol before being filtered, diluted, and succussed.
- POULTICE used in traditional medicine for the treatment of chilblains, infections, and arthritis.
- EATEN to thin and purify the blood and as an aid to clearing gastric and bronchial infections.

INDICATIONS

● NEURALGIA
Allium cepa is used to treat burning neuralgic pain that alternates from one side of the body to the other.

● COLDS & INFECTION
Onion causes the eyes and nose to water, and is used homeopathically to treat conditions that cause the same reaction in the body, such as influenza and colds. Antibiotic and antiseptic, it is also used to fight other forms of infection, such as of the chest or throat.

● HAY FEVER
Acute symptoms of hay fever, especially those accompanied by profuse watering of the eyes and irritating, burning catarrh, can be treated with *Allium cepa*. To be fully effective this may need to be taken in conjunction with other homeopathic remedies.

● CATARRH
Allium cepa eases the symptoms of watery catarrh, that burns the skin of the nose and the upper lip, causing it to become painful.

● POST-OPERATIVE
After amputation, many patients suffer from what is known as "phantom limb pain"; *Allium cepa* may be used as a pain-relieving treatment.

33

ALOE

Soothes grazes, scalds, and sunburn ◆ Calms varicose veins

Helps Irritable Bowel Syndrome and constipation

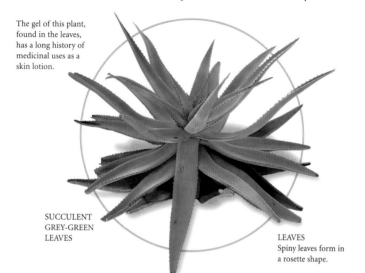

The gel of this plant, found in the leaves, has a long history of medicinal uses as a skin lotion.

SUCCULENT GREY-GREEN LEAVES

LEAVES
Spiny leaves form in a rosette shape.

KEY ACTIONS

- HEALS WOUNDS
- EMOLLIENT
- STIMULATES SECRETION OF BILE
- LAXATIVE

KEY PREPARATIONS

- BITTER ALOES The leaves exude a bitter liquid which is dried and known as 'bitter aloes'. This is used by herbalists to treat constipation.
- GEL Leaves are broken off and the clear gel is applied to the skin as a first aid remedy for burns.
- TINCTURE made from bitter aloes. Used to stimulate the appetite.

INDICATIONS

● **BEAUTY TREATMENT**
Aloe has a long history as a skin lotion – Cleopatra is said to have attributed her beauty to it.

● **FIRST AID**
Aloe is an excellent first aid remedy to keep in the home for burns, grazes, scalds, and sunburn. A leaf, broken off, releases soothing gel, which may be applied to the affected part.

● **LAXATIVE**
The bitter yellow liquid in the leaves (bitter aloes) are stongly laxative. They cause the colon to contract, generally producing a bowel movement 8–12 hours after consumption.

● **SKIN CONDITIONS**
The gel is useful for skin conditions that need soothing and astringing and will help varicose veins to some degree.

● **ULCERS**
The protective and healing effect of *Aloe* also works internally, and the gel can be used for peptic ulcers and irritable bowel syndrome.

● **CAUTION**
Do not use bitter aloes on the skin. Do not take during pregnancy. Do not take if suffering from haemorrhoids or kidney disease.

ALUMINA

Treats senile dementia and Alzheimer's disease

Alleviates fatigue ◆ Relieves constipation

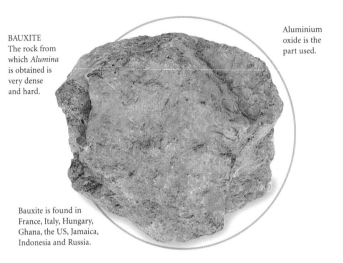

BAUXITE
The rock from which *Alumina* is obtained is very dense and hard.

Aluminium oxide is the part used.

Bauxite is found in France, Italy, Hungary, Ghana, the US, Jamaica, Indonesia and Russia.

KEY ACTIONS

- STIMULATES SLUGGISH BOWELS
- TREATS CONFUSION AND FAILING MEMORY
- EMOTIONALLY CALMING

KEY PREPARATIONS

- CRYSTALS of aluminium oxide are extracted from bauxite using an industrial process. They are then triturated with lactose sugar, filtered, diluted, and succussed.

INDICATIONS

● **DEMENTIA**
Alumina may be prescribed to help stem the alleviation of mental processes leading to sluggish and absent-minded behaviour, often associated with senile dementia and Alzheimer's disease. Elderly people are most commonly affected.

● **DIGESTION**
Traditionally used as an antacid in indigestion remedies, *Alumina* can also be found in food additives, baking powder, and drinking water.

● **CONSTIPATION**
There are different types of constipation; *Alumina* may be prescribed when a patient experiences difficulty with passing even soft stools.

● **NERVOUS DISORDERS**
Alumina is given to treat nervous complaints, particularly those characterized by a sense of muscle paralysis and fatigue. It may also be prescribed for delicate babies.

● **CAUTION**
Significant amounts of *Alumina* absorbed into the body are thought by some to cause the mental processes to slow down. Some evidence suggests that it may aid the development of Alzheimer's disease.

ANACARDIUM OCC.

Helps with exam nerves ◆ Soothes irritated skin

Effectively treats certain forms of depression

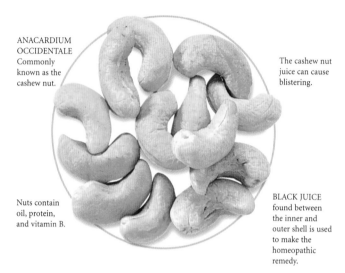

ANACARDIUM
OCCIDENTALE
Commonly
known as the
cashew nut.

The cashew nut
juice can cause
blistering.

Nuts contain
oil, protein,
and vitamin B.

BLACK JUICE
found between
the inner and
outer shell is used
to make the
homeopathic
remedy.

KEY ACTIONS

- REDUCES STRESS
- RELIEVES ANXIETY
- SOOTHING
- RELIEVES DEPRESSION

KEY PREPARATIONS

- TINCTURE made from the black juice found between the outer and inner shell of the cashew nut. It is dissolved in alcohol, then diluted and succussed.

INDICATIONS

● **EXAM NERVES**
Anacardium occ. is prescribed for extreme cases of anxiety about sitting exams. It assists with the student's feeling of inability to remember important revision. The treatment should be taken regularly before an exam. This remedy may also be effective when prescribed for performers suffering from stage fright.

● **DEPRESSION**
Depression associated with severe phobias, such as claustrophobia or agoraphobia, may be treated with *Anacardium occ.* This state, in common with severe

exam nerves (*see above*), may manifest itself in a lack of self-confidence and a worsening of eczema in sufferers.

● **SKIN CONDITIONS**
Anacardium occ. is prescribed for skin conditions that itch, burn, or swell and become sore, or for blisters that may become infected. It may also be prescribed for leprosy, and to treat warts.

● **CAUTION**
The juice of *Anacardium occ.* is an irritant which causes blistering if it comes into contact with the skin. In 19th-century Europe it was used medicinally to burn off warts and corns.

APIS

Relieves the swelling of hives ◆ Helps ease osteoarthritic pain ◆ Alleviates prostate problems

HONEY BEE
Carried only by the female bee, the sting can cause constriction of the airways or even collapse in people who are allergic to its poison.

One of the Apis remedy's main uses is to treat insect stings.

The Apis remedy is made from the whole bee, including the sting.

KEY ACTIONS

- PROVIDES RELIEF FROM ALLERGIES
- AIDS WITH FEELINGS OF JEALOUSY
- SOOTHES ANXIOUS RESTLESSNESS
- CURES CYSTITIS AND URINARY INFECTIONS

KEY PREPARATIONS

- TINCTURE made from the native European honey bee, which is now found in many parts of the world. The remedy is made from either the whole female bee, including the sting, or from the sting alone. The insect is crushed, dissolved in alcohol, diluted, and succussed.

INDICATIONS

● **PROSTATE PROBLEMS**
Prostitis (inflammation of the prostate) usually affects men in their thirties and forties; prostate cancer generally affects men over 60. *Apis* is indicated for an enlarged prostate with urine retention.

● **OSTEOARTHRITIS**
In some parts of the developed world up to 90 per cent of people over 40 have osteoarthritis. Severe osteoarthritis affects three times as many women as men. *Apis* is prescribed for inflammation of synovial membranes and overproduction of synovial fluids.

● **HIVES**
Also known as Urticaria, this condition consists of raised red patches – sometimes with paler centres – which itch intensely. It may be caused by food allergies, certain drugs, bites, stings, or stress. Treatment with *Apis* reduces the reaction.

● **ALLERGIES**
Apis is indicated as treatment for allergic swelling of the face, eyelids, lips, and mouth and other inflammation.

● **URINARY INFECTIONS**
Cystitis, oedema, and other urinary infections, including urine retention in newborn babies, can be treated with *Apis*.

ARGENTIUM NIT.

Prescribed for angina sufferers ◆ Eases Multiple Sclerosis

Relieves Irritable Bowel Syndrome

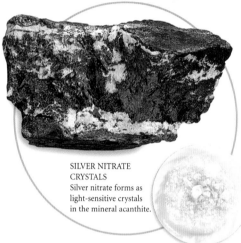

ACANTHITE
The mineral acanthite is the main ore of silver.

Acanthite is found in Norway, and North and South America.

SILVER NITRATE CRYSTALS
Silver nitrate forms as light-sensitive crystals in the mineral acanthite.

KEY ACTIONS

- CALMING
- CONTROLS THE INTESTINE
- USED TO TREAT WARTS
- AIDS THOSE WITH PHOBIAS

KEY PREPARATIONS

- TINCTURE made from pure crystals of silver nitrate dissolved in alcohol before being repeatedly diluted and succussed. *Argentum nit.* (silver nitrate) is found in acanthite, which usually occurs as crystals in hydrothermal veins in Norway, the US and South America.

INDICATIONS

● **PHOBIAS**
Sufferers of multiple phobias associated with anxiety neuroses that originate in previous experiences may benefit from *Argentum nit.*

● **IRRITABLE BOWEL SYNDROME (IBS)**
Argentum nit. is indicated for irritation of the mucous membranes of the intestine and control of the gut by the autonomic nervous system.

● **MULTIPLE SCLEROSIS**
MS occurs if the myelin sheaths surrounding nerve fibres are damaged. *Argentum nit.* has a direct,

qualitative effect upon nerves, controlling conscious movement.

● **ANGINA**
Argentum nit. is associated with improved nerve conduction to coronary arteries.

● **WARTS**
Argentum nit. was used for warts in the 19th century. It is still used in some wart medicines.

● **STRESS**
Argentum nit. is prescribed especially for exam stress.

● **CAUTION**
If ingested in large amounts, silver nitrate is highly poisonous.

ARNICA

Eases muscular pain, bruising, and sprains

Excellent first-aid remedy ◆ Helps control bleeding

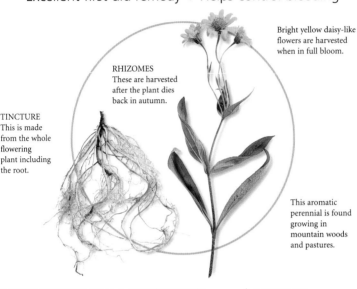

Bright yellow daisy-like flowers are harvested when in full bloom.

RHIZOMES
These are harvested after the plant dies back in autumn.

TINCTURE
This is made from the whole flowering plant including the root.

This aromatic perennial is found growing in mountain woods and pastures.

KEY ACTIONS

- PROMOTES TISSUE REPAIR
- ANTI-INFLAMMATORY
- TREATS GRIEF AND SHOCK
- EASES CRAMP

KEY PREPARATIONS

- OINTMENT used externally to improve local blood supply and speed healing in the treatment of bruises, sprains, and muscle pain.
- TINCTURE made from the whole flowering plant, including the root. It is steeped in alcohol, filtered, diluted, and succussed.

INDICATIONS

● SHOCK
Dizziness after a fall or injury can be treated with *Arnica*. It also treats the early stages of grief, when the person displays signs of shock.

● ERECTILE PROBLEMS
Arnica is given to treat erectile dysfunction caused by bruising.

● ANGINA
Arnica is prescribed to heal damaged heart muscle, such as after a heart attack.

● SKIN CONDITIONS
Eczema and cracked, blistered nipples can be treated with *Arnica*.

● FIRST AID
Arnica is given following an accident, surgery, bereavement, childbirth, or dental treatment.

● FEVER
Recurring fevers, such as occur with typhoid or malarial fever, can be treated with *Arnica*.

● CRAMP
Arnica relieves cramp. It is also prescribed for joint and muscular pain.

● CAUTION
Climbers used to chew, or drink an infusion of, *Arnica* leaves for aching muscles. Potentially toxic, its internal use is now mainly restricted to homeopathy.

BELLADONNA

Treats influenza and reduces fever ◆ Eases menstrual pains
Soothes painful, swollen breasts

FLOWERS
Purple, bell-shaped flowers give way to black berries in autumn.

LEAVES
Leaves have a weaker effect than the root, and for this reason are preferred for herbal medicines.

DEADLY NIGHTSHADE
Despite this plant's poisonous nature, it is used effectively in homeopathy.

KEY ACTIONS

- AIDS TEETHING INFANTS
- RELIEVES MASTITIS
- TREATS SUNSTROKE
- EASES KIDNEY PROBLEMS
- PRESCRIBED FOR ROSACEA

KEY PREPARATIONS

- TINCTURE made from the whole, fresh plant, including the root. As it comes into flower, the plant is dug up, chopped, and pounded to a pulp. The juice is then expressed and steeped in alcohol before being filtered, diluted, and succussed.

INDICATIONS

● TEETHING
Belladonna is prescribed to alleviate infant teething which is accompanied by sudden pain and a face that appears flushed.

● ROSACEA
Rosacea resembles mild adolescent acne. Its main feature is flushing of the skin. *Belladonna* is prescribed for the early stages, when the face is red, dry, and burning hot.

● WOMEN'S PROBLEMS
The remedy eases mastitis and menstrual pain.

● FEVER
Belladonna is a major remedy for acute illnesses of sudden violent onset. It treats febrile convulsions and sunstroke.

● ANAESTHETIC
Used in sleeping potions in Chaucer's time, today *Belladonna* provides an anaesthetic still used in conventional medicine.

● INFLUENZA
Influenza with high fever (dilated pupils, flushed skin, throbbing pain) is treated with *Belladonna*.

● KIDNEY PROBLEMS
Belladonna treats cystitis and nephritis (inflamed kidneys).

● CAUTION
Belladonna is poisonous if taken in large amounts.

Aurum Met.

Prescribed for gland cancer ◆ Alleviates certain causes
of infertility in men ◆ Treats circulatory problems

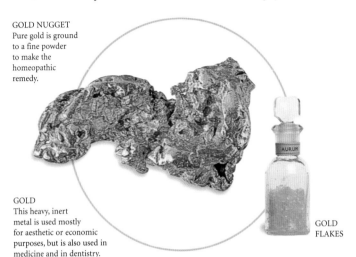

GOLD NUGGET
Pure gold is ground
to a fine powder
to make the
homeopathic
remedy.

GOLD
This heavy, inert
metal is used mostly
for aesthetic or economic
purposes, but is also used in
medicine and in dentistry.

**GOLD
FLAKES**

KEY ACTIONS

- HELPS WITH PHOBIAS
- TREATS REPRODUCTIVE
  DISORDERS
- CURES HEADACHES
- ALLEVIATES BONE PAINS
- PRESCRIBED FOR
  DEPRESSION AND GRIEF

KEY PREPARATIONS

- TINCTURE made from
  gold. The gold is
  purified from a
  nugget or extracted
  from an ore. It is
  then triturated with
  lactose sugar,
  filtered, diluted,
  and succussed.

INDICATIONS

● **CANCER**
There are many types of
cancer and, as such, as
wide a variety of
remedies. *Aurum met.* is
indicated for cancer of
the glands.

● **MALE INFERTILITY**
There are several causes
of male infertility, such as
malformation of the
testes or problems with
the testicles (vas
deferens). *Aurum met.*
treats childhood atrophy
of the testes and painful,
swollen testicles.

● **PHOBIAS**
Homeopaths examine the
physical symptoms that
accompany phobias

before prescribing a
specific remedy; *Aurum
met* is one indicated.

● **ARTHRITIS**
Aurum met. can help with
the treatment of
rheumatoid arthritis; a
condition whereby the
body's immune system
attacks the joints. The
remedy is indicated for
destruction of the bone.

● **CIRCULATION**
Aurum met. is prescribed
for circulatory problems,
such as palpitations and
angina.

● **CAUTION**
**If any palpitations are
severe, prolonged, or are
accompanied by chest
pains, consult a doctor.**

BARYTA CARB.

Assists in stroke victims' recovery ◆ Prescribed for
senile dementia ◆ Treats prostate problems and impotence

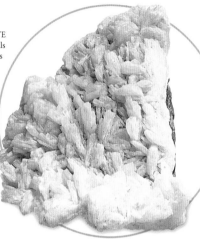

BARIUM
CARBONATE
White crystals
are odourless
and toxic.

WHITE CRYSTALS
of barite and witherite
are found together.

The crystals are
ground into
powder to make
the homeopathic
remedy.

Barium is an element
found in the earth's
crust in minerals
such as barite and
witherite.

KEY ACTIONS

- TREATS IMPOTENCE
- INDICATED FOR ANXIETY
  AND PHOBIAS
- USED FOR RECURRENT
  COLDS
- HELPS WITH DOWN'S
  SYNDROME
- PRESCRIBED FOR
  CONFUSION

KEY PREPARATIONS

- POWDER made from
  crystals of barium
  carbonate which
  have been chemically
  prepared (barium
  chloride precipitated
  with a weak solution
  of ammonia). The
  crystals are mixed
  with lactose sugar
  and triturated.

INDICATIONS

● **PROSTATE PROBLEMS**
Baryta carb. is prescribed
when the patient has a
frequent urge to urinate,
produces only a slow
stream of urine, or when
impotence occurs.

● **DEVELOPMENTAL
PROBLEMS**
The remedy is given for
senile dementia in the
elderly and for confusion.
It is also given for slow
physical or mental
development in children,
and for people with
Down's Syndrome.

● **STROKE**
Stroke occurs when the
blood supply to part of
the brain is interrupted or

insufficient. Strokes are
more likely to affect men
than women and
incidence rises sharply
with age. As symptoms
and sufferers vary, there
are several homeopathic
remedies for stroke.
Baryta carb. is suitable to
treat the very elderly and
the physically and
mentally weak.

● **COUGHS & COLDS**
Baryta carb. is indicated
for recurrent colds and
coughs, sore throats, and
swollen tonsils.

● **CAUTION**
Barium carbonate is a
powerful poison, used to
control rat populations.
It causes nausea and
vomiting if consumed.

BRYONIA

Eases painful breasts ◆ Alleviates constipation

Treats coughs and bronchitis

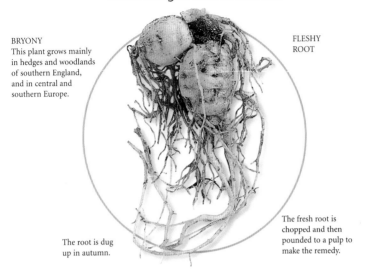

BRYONY
This plant grows mainly
in hedges and woodlands
of southern England,
and in central and
southern Europe.

FLESHY
ROOT

The fresh root is
chopped and then
pounded to a pulp to
make the remedy.

The root is dug
up in autumn.

KEY ACTIONS

• RELIEVES SORE BREASTS
• EASES CHEST PROBLEMS
• PAIN-RELIEVING
• ANTI-INFLAMMATORY

KEY PREPARATIONS

• TINCTURE made from
the fresh root. It is
unearthed before
the plant flowers,
chopped, pulped,
macerated in alcohol
for 10 days, diluted,
and succussed.

INDICATIONS

● PAIN RELIEF
The chief physical
symptom treated by
Bryonia is pain felt on the
slightest movement. This
includes bad headaches
and rheumatic pain.

● CONSTIPATION
Bryonia is indicated for
constipation where the
sufferer eventually passes
dry, hard stools and has
dry mucous membranes.

● CHEST PROBLEMS
Bryonia eases a variety of
chest problems, including
coughing accompanied by
chest pain or fever. It is
also prescribed to reduce
internal inflammation of
the chest, for pneumonia,

for shortness of breath,
and to clear phlegm.

● BRONCHITIS
Bryonia treats patients
suffering from bronchitis
which is accompanied by
a painful cough.

● BREAST PROBLEMS
For hard, inflamed
breasts, which are painful
on every movement (such
as before a period),
bryonia may be taken
regularly for up to a
maximum of five days.

● CAUTION
Used externally, the fresh
root of *Bryonia* can cause
severe skin irritation.
If ingested in excessive
amounts, it can cause
death within hours.

CALC. CARB.

Treats Chronic Fatigue Syndrome (CFS)

Prescribed for uterine fibroids ◆ Eases asthma

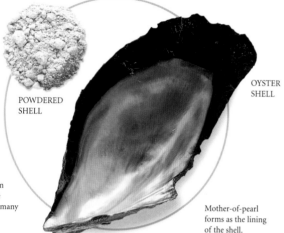

POWDERED
SHELL

OYSTER
SHELL

CALCIUM
CARBONATE
The homeopathic
remedy is made from
oyster shells, but the
calcified remains of many
crustaceans contain
calcium carbonate.

Mother-of-pearl
forms as the lining
of the shell.

KEY ACTIONS

- TREATS ECZEMA
- CALMS PALPITATIONS
- EASES ANXIETY
- PROMOTES GOOD
  DIGESTION
- HELPS WITH DENTAL
  PROBLEMS
- RELIEVES HEADACHES

KEY PREPARATIONS

- POWDERED SHELL
  made from mother-
  of-pearl, secreted by
  oysters. The mother-
  of-pearl is removed
  from the outer shell.
  It is cleaned, dried,
  and triturated with
  lactose sugar.

INDICATIONS

● **ANXIETY**
Calc. carb. is prescribed
for anxiety-related
conditions and phobias,
particularly those that
may escalate into
obsessive behaviour.

● **ECZEMA**
The cause of eczema is
often unknown and
symptoms vary. The
homeopath will want to
know a full medical
history, including that of
the patient's family, and
any possible triggers. *Calc.
carb.* is one remedy given.

● **CHEST PROBLEMS**
Asthma, and other
ailments arising out of
restricted movement of

the ribcage, are treated
with *Calc. carb.*

● **PALPITATIONS**
Not all palpitations are
serious, but they should
always be investigated by
a doctor. *Calc. carb.* is
among several remedies
recommended by
homeopaths.

● **CHRONIC FATIGUE
SYNDROME (CFS)**
Calc. carb. treats fatigue,
particularly of the thigh
muscles, from walking.

● **FIBROIDS**
Fibroids are benign (non-
cancerous) tumours. *Calc.
carb.* is used for the
treatment of growths on
stalks that project from
the uterine wall.

CALC. PHOS.

Relieves painful breasts ◆ Maintains strong bones

Prescribed for rheumatoid arthritis

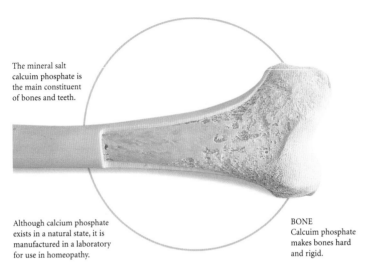

The mineral salt calcium phosphate is the main constituent of bones and teeth.

Although calcium phosphate exists in a natural state, it is manufactured in a laboratory for use in homeopathy.

BONE
Calcium phosphate makes bones hard and rigid.

KEY ACTIONS

- TREATS ROSACEA
- PRESCRIBED FOR PHOBIAS
- EASES TEETHING PROBLEMS
- PROMOTES GOOD DIGESTION

KEY PREPARATIONS

- MINERAL SALTS made from white calcium phosphate precipitate. It is filtered, dried, and triturated with lactose sugar.

INDICATIONS

● BONES
Calcium and phosphorus are essential to bone maintenance. *Calc. phos.* treats conditions such as slow-healing fractures, joint disorders, and slow growth in children.

● DIGESTIVE DISORDERS
Calc. phos. promotes good digestion in those who find it difficult to eat, due perhaps to cramps, pain, nausea, or diarrhoea.

● ARTHRITIS
This remedy is used to treat rheumatoid arthritis. *Calc. phos.* affects the maintenance of bones and is given if they are soft, thin, and brittle.

● ROSACEA
Calc. phos. is prescribed for rosacea that is found mainly on the nose, and is accompanied by pimples.

● PHOBIAS
There are many types of phobia; *Calc. phos.* is often used to treat those centred around school.

● BREAST PROBLEMS
Calc. phos. is given for painful breast lumps and swelling.

● TEETH
Teething problems and weak teeth are treated with *Calc. phos.*

● FATIGUE
Calc. phos. is indicated for fatigue and anaemia.

45

CANTHARIS

Key treatment for intestinal disorders

Treats kidney problems ◆ Eases cystitis

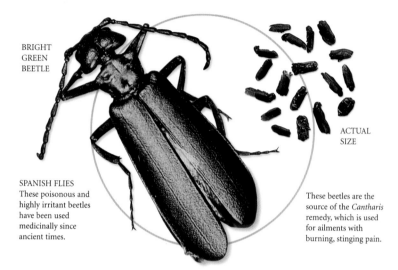

BRIGHT
GREEN
BEETLE

ACTUAL
SIZE

SPANISH FLIES
These poisonous and
highly irritant beetles
have been used
medicinally since
ancient times.

These beetles are the
source of the *Cantharis*
remedy, which is used
for ailments with
burning, stinging pain.

KEY ACTIONS

- PAIN-RELIEVING
- ANTI-INFLAMMATORY
- CONTROLS EXCESSIVE
  LIBIDO
- TREATS URINARY
  DISORDERS
- PROMOTES GOOD
  DIGESTION

KEY PREPARATIONS

- TINCTURE made from
  whole, live beetles.
  They are killed by
  heating, macerated
  in alcohol, and left
  to stand for 5 days.
  They are then
  filtered, diluted, and
  succussed.

INDICATIONS

● **KIDNEYS**
Cantharis is given for
tenderness in the kidneys,
for renal colic, and kidney
inflammation.

● **ULCERATIVE COLITIS**
Ulcerative colitis is an
inflammatory bowel
disease in which the
linings of the rectum and
colon gradually become
more ulcerated. *Cantharis*
reduces inflammation of
the gut lining and the
production of mucus.

● **EXCESSIVE LIBIDO**
Often claimed as
aphrodisiac, *Cantharis* is
given for uncontrollable,
inappropriate sexual
arousal.

● **CYSTITIS**
Cystitis affects mainly
women, but can be
present in men. Regular
doses of *Cantharis* are
prescribed. The remedy
also treats urinary tract
inflammation.

● **IRRITABLE BOWEL
SYNDROME (IBS)**
Inflammation of the
gastrointestinal tract,
especially the lower bowel,
is treated with *Cantharis*.

● **CAUTION**
This beetle secretes
cantharidine if touched.
This active chemical
causes the skin to blister
and, if ingested in large
quantities, is a powerful
poison that attcks the
urinary system.

CARBO VEG.

Alleviates symptoms of Chronic Fatigue Syndrome (CFS)

Eases indigestion ◆ Reduces bloating

Woods from different trees make charcoal with different properties. Silver birch, beech or poplar trees are used in homepathy.

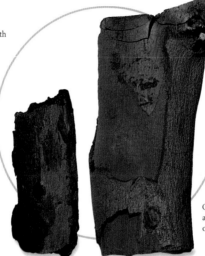

CHARCOAL
Wood is burnt in a sealed environment from which air is excluded to make charcoal.

Charcoal is very hard and does not rot like ordinary wood.

KEY ACTIONS

- RELIEVES FLATULENCE
- TREATS FATIGUE
- A PURIFIER
- ANTISEPTIC
- IMPROVES CIRCULATION
- AIDS BREATHING

KEY PREPARATIONS

- TINCTURE made from the wood of the silver birch, beech, or poplar trees. Fist-sized bits of wood are cut, heated until red hot, and sealed in an airtight earthenware jar. The resulting ash is then triturated, diluted, and succussed.

INDICATIONS

● **CHRONIC FATIGUE SYNDROME (CFS)**
Carbo veg. alleviates aches and burning pains all over the body, as well as confusion, bloating, flatulence, and fainting.

● **BLOATING**
Bloating and flatulence may be due to constipation or intestinal problems. If the condition is relieved by burping, a homeopath may recommend *Carbo veg.*

● **INDIGESTION**
For indigestion with excessive flatulence, especially that which occurs regardless of the patient's diet, *Carbo veg.*

should be taken regularly. It is also prescribed for those with a poor, sluggish constitution, particularly elderly patients.

● **ANTISEPTIC**
Used throughout history as a "purifier". In the 18th and 19th centuries *Carbo veg.* was used in dressings for ulcers and in some mouthwashes. It is used in both traditional and conventional medicine for ulceration and septic diseases, and is known for its deodorant and disinfectant properties.

● **BREATHING TROUBLE**
Used to treat spasmodic coughs, whooping cough, asthma, and bronchitis in the elderly.

CAUSTICUM

Prescribed for weakness in the nerves or muscles

Cures bed-wetting ◆ Treats warts and veruccas

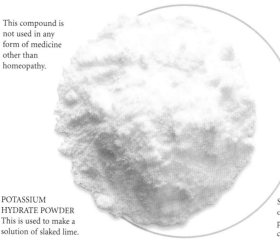

This compound is not used in any form of medicine other than homeopathy.

POTASSIUM HYDRATE POWDER
This is used to make a solution of slaked lime.

Slaked lime and sulphate of potash are dissolved in purified water to make the causticum tincture.

KEY ACTIONS

- MAJOR FIRST AID REMEDY
- TREATS BELL'S PALSY AND MULTIPLE SCLEROSIS
- PROMOTES SKIN HEALING
- CURES LARYNGITIS

KEY PREPARATIONS

- TINCTURE made from slaked lime and sulphate of potash. They are combined and dissolved in purified water. This solution is then further diluted and succussed.

INDICATIONS

● **MULTIPLE SCLEROSIS**
Causticum is indicated for progressive debilitation of the nervous system.

● **MUSCLE WEAKNESS**
Causticum is most often prescribed for weakness, which may progress to paralysis, of the nerves and muscles, especially of the bladder, larynx, vocal cords, upper eyelids, and the right side of the face. Muscle weakness may show both as twitching and as stiffness that causes mobility problems.

● **WARTS**
For veruccas or warts that occur near the nails, or on the face or eyelids, a

course of *Causticum*, lasting for approximately three weeks, may be given.

● **FIRST AID**
Causticum is a first aid remedy for severe burns.

● **SKIN CONDITIONS**
Slow-healing burns, scars, and blisters, as well as boils, eczema, herpes, and acne may benefit from using *Causticum*.

● **LARYNGITIS**
Use *Causticum* for laryngitis with a dry, raw throat and violent cough.

● **BED-WETTING**
Causticum, taken before bed, cures bed-wetting that occurs soon after the patient falls asleep.

IPECAC.

Prescribed for morning sickness ◆ Stems heavy

menstrual bleeding ◆ Alleviates general nausea

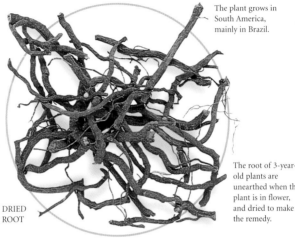

The plant grows in South America, mainly in Brazil.

IPECACUANHA
A traditional Brazilian cure for dysentery that was brought to Europe in 1672, and is still used today by herbalists for amoebic dysentery.

The root of 3-year-old plants are unearthed when the plant is in flower, and dried to make the remedy.

DRIED ROOT

KEY ACTIONS

- EASES WHEEZING AND ASTHMA
- TREATS NOSEBLEEDS
- PRESCRIBED FOR COUGHS
- USED TO STOP HEAVY BLEEDING

KEY PREPARATIONS

- TINCTURE made from the root. It is dug up and the firmest, darkest rootlets are dried, powdered, and macerated in alcohol. They are then filtered, diluted, and succussed.

INDICATIONS

● **NAUSEA**
Persistent nausea, with or without vomiting, is treated with *Ipecac.* For constant nausea, possibly accompanied by headaches, perspiration, and diarrhoea, *Ipecac.* should be taken regularly.

● **ASTHMA**
The remedy is prescribed for patients whose asthma attacks are accompanied by persistent nausea.

● **COUGHS & WHEEZING**
Ipecac. is prescribed for coughing fits which cause wheezing, breathing difficulties, and a constricted chest. It is effective in treating

irritating, dry, rattling loose coughs, and those triggered by warm or humid weather.

● **MORNING SICKNESS**
Ipecac. may be prescribed for morning sickness where, despite vomiting, the tongue remains clean and unfurred.

● **BLEEDING**
Ipecac. is prescribed to treat nosebleeds and heavy menstrual bleeding. It is also given to patients with a general tendency to bleed easily.

● **CAUTION**
In large doses, *Ipecac.* causes nausea and vomiting; it may also lead to cardiac failure.

CHAMOMILLA

Cures sleeplessness ◆ Calms irritability in children
and adults ◆ Treats toothache and earache

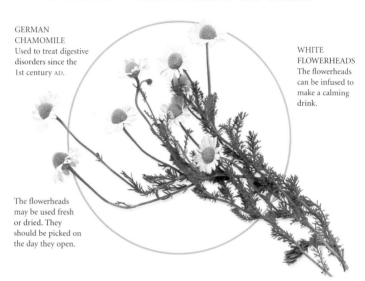

GERMAN
CHAMOMILE
Used to treat digestive
disorders since the
1st century AD.

WHITE
FLOWERHEADS
The flowerheads
can be infused to
make a calming
drink.

The flowerheads
may be used fresh
or dried. They
should be picked on
the day they open.

KEY ACTIONS

- CALMING
- SOOTHING
- PAIN-RELIEVING
- ASSISTS WITH LABOUR
  AND MENSTRUAL PAINS

KEY PREPARATIONS

- INFUSION made from
  the flowerheads. It is
  well known as a
  calming drink.
- OIL made from the
  flower heads. Used
  to treat hay fever
  and asthma.
- TINCTURE made from
  the whole, fresh
  plant, harvested
  when in flower. It is
  finely chopped and
  macerated in alcohol
  before being diluted,
  and succussed.

INDICATIONS

● **CHILDREN'S HEALTH**
Chamomilla is often given
to children who are
snappy, wail when ill, and
are pacified only by being
held. It is prescribed for
teething with irritability
and anger, and for temper
tantrums when the child
is impossible to please.

● **TOOTHACHE**
Toothache accompanied
by unbearable pain, such
as when an abscess occurs,
can be treated with
Chamomilla.

● **PAIN RELIEF**
Chamomilla provides
relief from pain which
seems unbearable.
Symptoms it can alleviate

include: excruciating
earache accompanied by
fever, stomach pain with
diarrhoea, colic, and
swollen glands causing
facial and neck pain.

● **WOMEN'S HEALTH**
Women's health problems
alleviated by *Chamomilla*
include menstrual pains
which induce sweats,
anger, or fainting; labour
pains; inflamed nipples;
and pain from breast-
feeding, causing anger in
the mother.

● **SLEEPLESSNESS**
A course of *Chamomilla*
reduces sleeplessness
caused by anger and
irritability. Drinking
chamomile tea before bed
also promotes good sleep.

CHELIDONIUM

Treats liver problems, including hepatitis ◆ Used in pre-operative care ◆ Prescribed for lung complaints

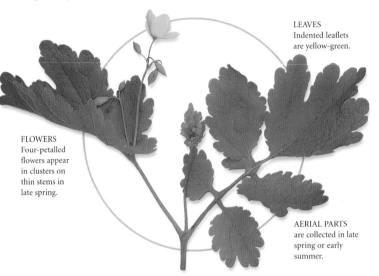

LEAVES
Indented leaflets are yellow-green.

FLOWERS
Four-petalled flowers appear in clusters on thin stems in late spring.

AERIAL PARTS
are collected in late spring or early summer.

KEY ACTIONS

- ANTI-SPASMODIC
- PAIN-RELIEVING
- TREATS GALLSTONES
- USED FOR PNEUMONIA

KEY PREPARATIONS

- SAP The freshly crushed plant exudes a sticky orange sap, which herbalists use to treat warts and corns.
- TINCTURE made from either the whole flowering plant, or just the root. It is chopped, pulped, and macerated in alcohol for at least 10 days.

INDICATIONS

● **PRE-OPERATIVE CARE**
Chelidonium may be given prior to surgery linked to hepatitis or gallstones.

● **LIVER PROBLEMS**
Chelidonium is associated with liver problems, as well as those arising from the spleen, kidney, and intestine. It is effective in treating hepatitis.

● **GALL-BLADDER**
This remedy is used in traditional medicine for problems arising from the gall-bladder. Patients with gallstones feel pain on the upper right side of the abdomen – *Chelidonium* is associated with right-sided symptoms.

● **PAIN RELIEF**
Chelidonium is a muscle relaxant and, as such, useful for relieving pain, such as headaches which occur on the right side of the head, backache, and shoulder pain.

● **LUNGS**
Pneumonia, especially that which chiefly affects the right lung, and other lung complaints may be treated with *Chelidonium*.

● **EYES**
Dioscorides, the famous Greek physician from the 1st century AD, prescribed *Chelidonium* for eye problems and to sharpen the eyesight. Western and Chinese herbalists use it to treat cataracts.

CHINA

Key treatment for malaria ◆ Relieves Chronic Fatigue Syndrome (CFS) ◆ Treats exhaustion

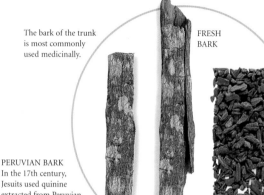

The bark of the trunk is most commonly used medicinally.

FRESH BARK

PERUVIAN BARK
In the 17th century, Jesuits used quinine extracted from Peruvian bark, as a cure for malaria. It was widely adopted in Europe as a treatment for fevers.

DRIED BARK

KEY ACTIONS

- RELIEVES INSOMNIA
- HELPS REPLENISH LOST FLUIDS
- TREATS FEVER
- EASES HEADACHES
- PRESCRIBED FOR INDIGESTION

KEY PREPARATIONS

- TINCTURE made from dried Peruvian bark. It is macerated in alcohol for at least five days, before being filtered, diluted, and then succussed.

INDICATIONS

● MALARIA
This bark is of particular historical significance for homeopaths, since quinine extracted from it became the subject of Hahnemann's first homeopathic proving. Today the remedy is a key treatment for malarial symptoms.

● HEADACHES
China treats throbbing pains in the head, possibly linked to facial neuralgia, nosebleeds, tinnitus, or liver disorders.

● CHRONIC FATIGUE SYNDROME (CFS)
China is prescribed to CFS sufferers to help combat bloating, anxiety, sleeplessness, and a feeling of weakness after the slightest exertion.

● EXHAUSTION
The remedy is used for exhaustion following illness or extreme fluid loss.

● INSOMNIA
Sleeplessness due to excited thoughts, where even the slightest noise disrupts the sleeper, can be treated with *China*.

● CAUTION
The bark of this tropical tree yields quinine, which, if taken in large doses, causes harmful symptoms similar to those of malaria.

COFFEA

Used in painkillers ◆ Treats insomnia

Cures headaches and toothache

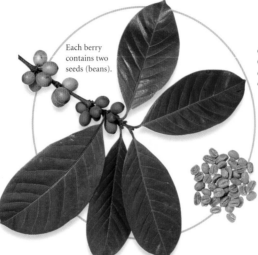

Each berry contains two seeds (beans).

COFFEE
Coffee's stimulating effect is weakened if drunk repeatedly.

COFFEE BEANS
The best quality beans are produced by fermenting, sun-drying, and roasting seeds.

KEY ACTIONS

- CURES PALPITATIONS
- REDUCES OVER-EXCITEMENT
- RELIEVES MENOPAUSAL FLUSHES
- PAIN-RELIEVING

KEY PREPARATIONS

- BERRIES The raw berries were originally chewed as a stimulant.
- TINCTURE made from ripe, unroasted coffee beans. These are macerated in alcohol for at least five days before being filtered. The resulting liquid is then repeatedly diluted and succussed.

INDICATIONS

● **PAIN RELIEF**
In modern medicine, caffeine is combined with conventional analgesics, such as aspirin, to make over-the-counter painkillers. *Coffea* is recommended for hypersensitivity to pain, to the point where pain causes intense despair.

● **INSOMNIA**
Coffea can help combat insomnia, particularly that which derives from an inability to relax.

● **HEADACHES**
Coffea is prescribed for one-sided pain in the head which feels as if a nail is being driven into it, and for pain that sets in upon waking and can seem unbearable. Ayurvedic medicine uses unripe beans to treat headaches.

● **TOOTHACHE**
For toothache with severe, shooting pain – that often shoots from the teeth to the tips of the fingers – take *Coffea* daily.

● **OVEREXCITEMENT**
Coffea is prescribed to reduce overexcitement and calm palpitations.

● **CAUTION**
Excessive consumption of caffeine upsets digestion, drains the body of calcium, and can cause nervousness.

CONIUM

Prescribed for cancer ◆ Treats prostate problems ◆ Relieves breast pain

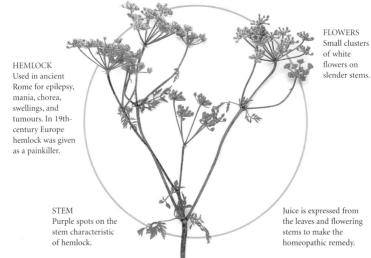

HEMLOCK
Used in ancient Rome for epilepsy, mania, chorea, swellings, and tumours. In 19th-century Europe hemlock was given as a painkiller.

FLOWERS
Small clusters of white flowers on slender stems.

STEM
Purple spots on the stem characteristic of hemlock.

Juice is expressed from the leaves and flowering stems to make the homeopathic remedy.

KEY ACTIONS

- COUNTERS PREMATURE AGEING
- TREATS CYSTS
- RELIEVES MENTAL STRAIN
- RESTORES VITALITY

KEY PREPARATIONS

- TINCTURE made from the fresh flowering plant, including the root. It is macerated in alcohol, diluted, and succussed.

INDICATIONS

● **TUMOURS**
Breast lumps mainly occur in women aged between 30 and 50; 80 per cent are benign, but all should be investigated by a doctor. Hard breast tumours are treated with *Conium* – it was used for breast tumours in the 1st century AD. It is also indicated for treatment of tumours or cysts in the reproductive organs.

● **MENTAL STRAIN**
Conium treats illnesses caused by mental strain or grief.

● **PROSTATE PROBLEMS**
Conium is given for an enlarged prostate, particularly when a discharge of prostatic fluid occurs.

● **BREAST PAIN**
Conium is prescribed for breast pain, especially that which occurs when the breast is tender even when touched lightly.

● **THE ELDERLY**
In the elderly, *Conium* is thought to restore vitality; it is also believed to counter premature ageing.

● **CAUTION**
The toxins in this plant can cause paralysis, primarily of the respiratory nerves. This leads to death by suffocation if *Conium* is taken in excess.

COLOCYNTHIS

Prescribed for Irritable Bowel Syndrome

Treats gastroenteritis ◆ Relieves sciatica

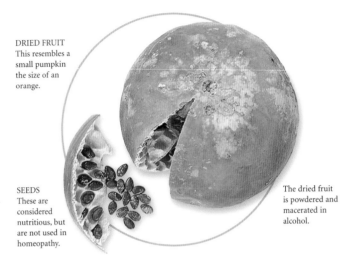

DRIED FRUIT
This resembles a
small pumpkin
the size of an
orange.

SEEDS
These are
considered
nutritious, but
are not used in
homeopathy.

The dried fruit
is powdered and
macerated in
alcohol.

KEY ACTIONS

- PAIN-RELIEVING
- TREATS ULCERATIVE COLITIS
- RELIEVES SCIATICA
- CURES COLIC

KEY PREPARATIONS

- TINCTURE made from the dried, deseeded fruit. It is powdered and then macerated in alcohol before being diluted and succussed.

INDICATIONS

● PAIN RELIEF

Colocynthis is given for the relief of acute pain and especially for: colicky abdominal pain; cramping in the hips, kidneys, and ovaries; headaches; or shooting nerve pain in the face, neck, and limbs. It may also be prescribed for gout and for rheumatic pain in the neck.

● GASTROENTERITIS

Gastroenteritis where the patient suffers severe abdominal cramps can be treated with *Colocynthis*.

● SCIATICA

There are several homeopathic remedies for different forms of sciatica. *Colocynthis* treats that which worsens in cold, damp weather.

● IRRITABLE BOWEL SYNDROME (IBS)

The remedy treats griping pains that are relieved when the patient bends double or applies pressure to the abdomen.

● COLIC

Colocynthis is indicated for colic with severe pains.

● CAUTION

Colocynthis is a bitter gourd which contains a substance called colocynthin. It causes severe cramps and gastrointestinal inflammation if ingested.

CUPRUM MET.

Cures cramp in the extremities and stomach

Eases physical and mental exhaustion ◆ Treats convulsions

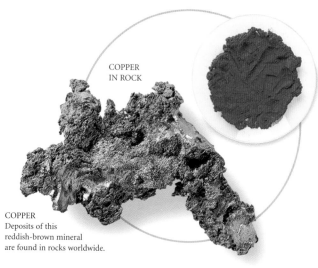

COPPER
IN ROCK

POWDERED
COPPER
Copper is
powdered to
make the
homeopathic
remedy.

COPPER
Deposits of this
reddish-brown mineral
are found in rocks worldwide.

KEY ACTIONS

- ANTI-SPASMODIC
- PAIN-RELIEVING
- ALLEVIATES COLICKY
  CONDITIONS

KEY PREPARATIONS

- TINCTURE made
  from powdered
  copper. The metal
  is triturated with
  lactose sugar, then
  ground repeatedly
  until it forms
  a water-soluble
  powder. It is
  filtered, diluted,
  and succussed.
- TRACE ELEMENT
  found in many
  foods. It is vital for
  maintaining a
  healthy body and for
  good bone growth.

INDICATIONS

● **CRAMP**
This occurs when the
muscles go into spasm as
a result of shortage of
oxygen or from a build-
up of lactic acid. *Cuprum
met.* is indicated primarily
for severe cramp in the
legs, fingers, or feet.

● **CONVULSIONS**
Cuprum met. is given for
convulsions, including
those linked to epilepsy
and those experienced by
very young children.

● **EXHAUSTION**
The remedy is prescribed
to relieve exhaustion,
perhaps following illness,
lack of sleep, or severe
mental strain. Symptoms

may include cramps and
headaches between the
eyes. The remedy is linked
to the nervous system.

● **DIGESTION**
Cuprum met. is chiefly
associated with the
digestive system,
especially with alleviating
stomach cramps. It is
effective in easing
spasmodic, colicky pains,
and when the abdomen is
hot, tender, and sore.

● **CAUTION**
Although used by
doctors as late as the
1880s in ointments for
healing wounds, copper
is toxic. Acute copper
poisoning can cause
convulsions, paralysis,
and even death.

STAPHYSAGRIA

Treats urogenital problems ◆ Cures insomnia

Relieves headaches and toothache

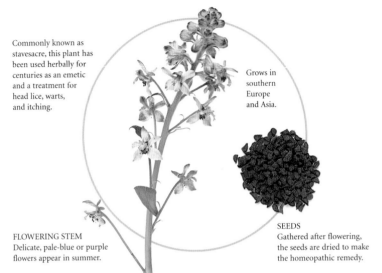

Commonly known as stavesacre, this plant has been used herbally for centuries as an emetic and a treatment for head lice, warts, and itching.

Grows in southern Europe and Asia.

FLOWERING STEM
Delicate, pale-blue or purple flowers appear in summer.

SEEDS
Gathered after flowering, the seeds are dried to make the homeopathic remedy.

KEY ACTIONS

- CALMS PALPITATIONS
- TREATS PAINFUL SKIN CONDITIONS
- SOOTHES SORE EYES
- USED FOR GRIEF
- INDICATED FOR INFERTILITY IN WOMEN

KEY PREPARATIONS

- OINTMENT Used to treat head lice and other parasites.
- POWDER The seeds of the plant are gathered once it has finished flowering. They are dried, triturated, and succussed.

INDICATIONS

● **INFERTILITY**
Provided there are no physiological problems, constitutional treatment will try to rectify imbalances in the body systems controlling reproduction. Remedies are determined largely by an individual's symptoms. *Staphisagria* is associated with women.

● **GRIEF**
Staphisagria is indicated for suppressed grief, linked to embarrassment or humiliation.

● **SKIN CONDITIONS**
Staphisagria is used to treat skin conditions that are affected by irritability

of the nervous system, such as psoriasis.

● **VAGINISMUS**
An unusual condition in which the muscles surrounding the entrance of the vagina go into spasm, making sexual intercourse, medical examination, or the use of tampons painful or impossible. *Staphisagria* is prescribed for vaginismus which occurs after medical examination.

● **EYES**
The remedy soothes inflamed, painful eyes, and treats styes.

● **CAUTION**
The seeds of *Staphisagria* are a powerful poison.

DIOSCOREA

Treats menstrual problems ◆ Prescribed for renal colic

and kidney stones ◆ Key remedy for severe pains

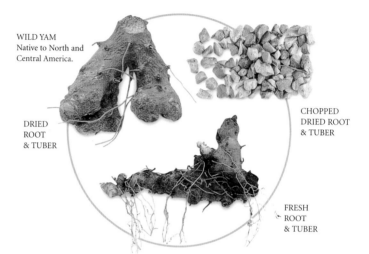

WILD YAM
Native to North and
Central America.

DRIED
ROOT
& TUBER

CHOPPED
DRIED ROOT
& TUBER

FRESH
ROOT
& TUBER

KEY ACTIONS

- PAIN-RELIEVING
- TREATS NEURALGIA
- PRESCRIBED FOR COLIC
- ALLEVIATES LIVER
  PROBLEMS

KEY PREPARATIONS

- TINCTURE made from
  the fresh root, dug
  up after the plant
  has flowered. It is
  chopped and
  macerated in alcohol.

INDICATIONS

● **COLIC**
Dioscorea (wild yam), a
traditional Aztec remedy
for pain, was used in
Central America for colic.
Today it is prescribed for
colicky pains, and for
neuralgic pains of the
gastrointestinal system.

● **WOMEN'S HEALTH**
Used by the Aztecs for
menstrual pain, and still
given for menstruation
problems. *Dioscorea* was
also used in production of
the first contraceptive pill.

● **MEN'S HEALTH**
In men, *Dioscorea* is
typically prescribed to
treat renal colic associated
with kidney stones, sharp

pains radiating down the
testicles and legs, and
where cold, clammy
perspiration is present.

● **PAIN RELIEF**
Dioscorea is indicated for
pains that are typically
severe, cutting, cramping,
and grinding, and for
those that radiate out in
all directions from a
central point, which may
shift in location. The
pains may affect the area
of the liver, and radiate
upwards in the direction
of the right nipple.

● **CAUTION**
Wild yam should not be
taken without medical
advice by women who
are also taking the
contraceptive pill.

EUPHRASIA

Soothes conjunctivitis ◆ Eases general eye problems

Treats hay fever and other allergies

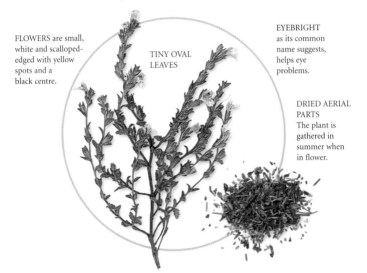

FLOWERS are small, white and scalloped-edged with yellow spots and a black centre.

TINY OVAL LEAVES

EYEBRIGHT as its common name suggests, helps eye problems.

DRIED AERIAL PARTS The plant is gathered in summer when in flower.

KEY ACTIONS

- ANTI-INFLAMMATORY
- SOOTHES IRRITATION
- REDUCES EYE STRAIN
- TREATS ALLERGIES

KEY PREPARATIONS

- EYEWASH Bathe your eyes with *Euphrasia* solution: 2 drops of the mother tincture added to a saltwater eyebath – 5 ml/1 tsp salt to 150 ml/5 fl oz boiled, cooled water.
- TINCTURE made from the whole, fresh flowering plant, including the root. It is chopped and macerated in alcohol.

INDICATIONS

● ALLERGIES

The remedy is used mainly for allergies and infection affecting the eyes and nose, such as colds and hay fever, where the eyes are mainly affected. It is also indicated for allergies affecting the middle ear and sinuses.

● EYE PROBLEMS

Also known as eyebright, *Euphrasia* has a classic affinity to the eyes. It has been used to treat eye strain and inflammation since the Middle Ages. Today it is given for irritation with cutting, burning, pressing pains and sticky mucus; when eyes have a heightened sensitivity to light, with burning, swollen eyelids and frequent blinking; and when eyes water profusely. It may also be prescribed for eye symptoms which occur after an injury.

● CONJUNCTIVITIS

Inflammation of the conjunctiva results either from infection (yellow discharge) or allergy (whites of the eyes are red and gritty). Conjunctivitis is typified by the presence of swollen eyelids with a burning discharge and a frequent need to blink. In some cases, little blisters may form inside the eyelids. *Euphrasia* is the usual remedy prescribed.

SPONGIA

Treats heart problems ◆ Eases respiratory trouble

Prescribed for certain phobias

FRESH SPONGE
is roasted to make
a remedy for
swelling of the
thyroid glands
and coughs.

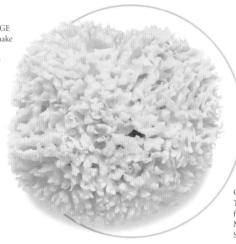

COMMON SPONGE
Traditionally gathered
from the waters of the
Mediterranean, near
Syria and Greece.

KEY ACTIONS

- ANTI-INFLAMMATORY
- CALMING
- TREATS THYROID PROBLEMS
- FIGHTS INFECTION
- REDUCES PALPITATIONS

KEY PREPARATIONS

- POWDERED SPONGE
  The sponge is
  carefully cleaned of
  sand, then toasted in
  a metal drum before
  being powdered and
  triturated.

INDICATIONS

● **PHOBIAS**
Spongia (the common sponge) is appropriate for those who have a marked fear of heart disease and of death, particularly by suffocation. They may feel uncomfortable in clothes.

● **HEART PROBLEMS**
There is a strong focus on the heart with *Spongia.* Typical symptoms include palpitations or an uneasy feeling in the area of the heart. Congestion may result, with a sensation as though blood is rushing into the chest and face. A fear of suffocation and a sense of the heart being forced upwards can disrupt sleep. Other

symptoms include exhaustion and the body feeling heavy, so that even slight exertion causes prostration.

● **RESPIRATION**
Spongia is prescribed for upper-respiratory-tract infections that tend to settle in the larynx, such as a dry, hollow, croupy cough. There is typically a feeling of dryness in the mucous membranes, and pain in the larynx that worsens with swallowing, singing, or talking.

● **GLANDS**
Inflammation, hardening, and enlargement of the glands, especially the thyroid, can be treated effectively with *Spongia.*

FERRUM PHOS.

Treats urogenital problems ◆ Relieves digestive disorders

Assists sufferers of Raynaud's disease

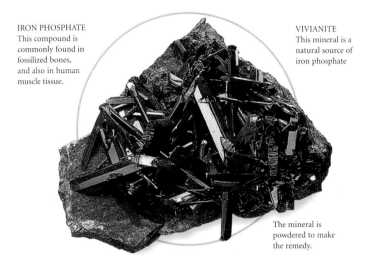

IRON PHOSPHATE
This compound is commonly found in fossilized bones, and also in human muscle tissue.

VIVIANITE
This mineral is a natural source of iron phosphate

The mineral is powdered to make the remedy.

KEY ACTIONS

- FIGHTS INFECTION
- IMPROVES CIRCULATION
- HELPS RESTORE MALE LIBIDO
- ANTI-INFLAMMATORY
- REDUCES FEVER

KEY PREPARATIONS

- TISSUE SALTS prepared chemically from iron sulphate, sodium phosphate, and sodium acetate. The powdered mineral is then triturated. Although it is chemically prepared for homeopathy, iron phosphate occurs naturally in vivianite.

INDICATIONS

● **COLDS**
Colds are caused by viral infections of the respiratory tract. A neglected cold may infect the chest, ears, throat, sinuses, or larynx. As such, it is important to treat the early signs of a cold. *Ferrum phos.* may be prescribed for a cold that comes on slowly.

● **FEVER**
Ferrum phos. fights infection at the early stages and reduces fever.

● **DIGESTIVE PROBLEMS**
Indigestion, sour burps, and vomiting of food that appears not to have been properly digested may be

treated with *Ferrum phos.* It may also be given for Irritable Bowel Syndrome or constipation.

● **MEN'S HEALTH**
Used to treat a marked loss of libido in men.

● **WOMEN'S HEALTH**
Ferrum phos. is used to treat dragging uterine pain, a short menstrual cycle, vaginal dryness, and nocturnal stress incontinence in women.

● **RAYNAUD'S DISEASE**
This is due to restricted blood flow when the blood vessels contract in the cold. *Ferrum phos.* is prescribed for this and other problems associated with poor circulation.

GELSEMIUM

Treats neurological disorders ◆ Reduces fever

Calms phobias and anticipatory fears

CAROLINA JASMINE
This came into regular
use from the middle of
the 19th century, chiefly
as a treatment for
nervous disorders,
such as sciatica and
neuralgia.

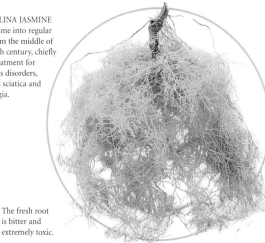

ROOTSTOCK
This is unearthed
in autumn, and
the aromatic fresh
root is used to
make homeopathic
remedies.

The fresh root
is bitter and
extremely toxic.

KEY ACTIONS

- CALMS STAGE FRIGHT
  AND EXAM NERVES
- TREATS SCIATICA
- EASES INFLUENZA
- HELPS HAY FEVER
  SUFFERERS

KEY PREPARATIONS

- TINCTURE made from
  the fresh bark of the
  root. It is finely
  chopped and
  macerated in alcohol.

INDICATIONS

● **FEARS**
Gelsemium is often used
to combat phobias, exam
nerves, stage fright, and
other anticipatory terrors.
At times the remedy has
been given to strengthen
courage on the battlefield.

● **NEUROLOGY**
A general state of physical
and/or mental paralysis,
with weakness and an
inability to perform, are
key symptoms linked to
this remedy. Certain
anticipatory terrors (*see
above*) cause trembling,
weakness, diarrhoea, and
frequent urination; in the
long term, these may lead
to more complicated
serious neurological

disorders, possibly even
paralysis, which the
remedy may help. It has
been used to treat
neuralgia, sciatica, and
other nervous disorders
since the middle of the
19th century.

● **INFLUENZA**
Gelsemium is used for
acute influenza. It eases
sore throats, limp limbs,
chills, fever (including
that accompanied by a
lack of thirst), headaches
with double vision, and
heavy, drooping eyelids.

● **HAY FEVER**
If accompanied by any of
the symptoms mentioned
under *Influenza*, hay fever
may be treated effectively
with *Gelsemium*.

GRAPHITES

Treats glandular disorders ◆ Soothes irritated, cracked,

and infected skin ◆ Eases painful periods

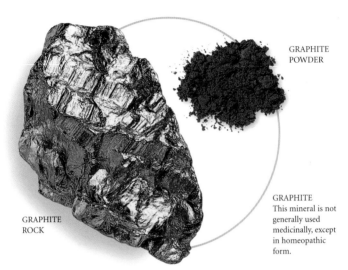

GRAPHITE
POWDER

GRAPHITE
ROCK

GRAPHITE
This mineral is not
generally used
medicinally, except
in homeopathic
form.

KEY ACTIONS

- AIDS DIGESTION
- EASES PAINFUL BREASTS
- RELIEVES CONSTIPATION, BLOATING, AND FLATULENCE
- TREATS UROGENITARY DISORDERS

KEY PREPARATIONS

- TINCTURE made from graphite powder. It is triturated with lactose sugar to make it soluble. After being dissolved in water it is repeatedly diluted and succussed.

INDICATIONS

● **ERECTILE PROBLEMS**
Graphites is effective for impotence in men with a high libido at an early age. It is also prescribed for priapism (persistent, sore erection).

● **MENSTRUATION**
Irregular, scanty periods and swollen, hard, painful breasts before and during menstruation can be eased with this remedy. It also treats itchy genitals and constipation during menstruation.

● **SKIN CONDITIONS**
Irritated skin, eczema, psoriasis, and cracked skin may be alleviated with *Graphites*. As may ill-

conditioned nails. The remedy is also effective for painful scars, cold sores, and genital herpes.

● **DIGESTIVE PROBLEMS**
Graphites is given for constipation, bloating, and flatulence. It is also effective for anal fissures, haemorrhoids, rectal itching, and stomach pains with hunger or vomiting.

● **GLANDS**
Graphites is commonly prescribed for physical symptoms which tend to affect the left side of the body and are often linked to glandular problems. Sensitivity to the cold and headaches after skipping meals are also typical.

HAMAMELIS

Treats varicose veins ◆ Prescribed for haemorrhoids
Useful first aid remedy

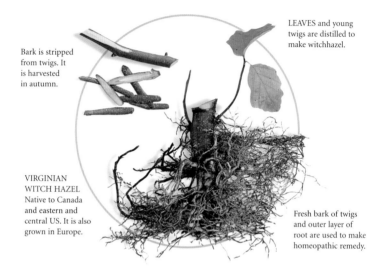

Bark is stripped from twigs. It is harvested in autumn.

LEAVES and young twigs are distilled to make witchhazel.

VIRGINIAN WITCH HAZEL Native to Canada and eastern and central US. It is also grown in Europe.

Fresh bark of twigs and outer layer of root are used to make homeopathic remedy.

KEY ACTIONS

- EASES HEAVY PERIODS
- ASTRINGENT
- ANTI-INFLAMMATORY

KEY PREPARATIONS

- POULTICE used by Native Americans for tumours and inflammation.
- TINCTURE made from fresh chopped bark taken from the twigs and roots, steeped in alcohol.
- SUPPOSITORIES used for haemorrhoids.

INDICATIONS

● **VARICOSE VEINS**
This condition is caused when the valves inside the veins start to fail and blood pools form. They appear as twisted, purple lines, mainly affecting the legs. *Hamamelis* is prescribed for varicose veins with a sore, bruised feeling. Varicose veins may be hereditary, or may result from pregnancy, obesity, or thrombosis.

● **HAEMORRHOIDS**
Haemorrhoids, also known as "piles", are swollen veins in the lower rectum and around the anus. They are often due to constipation, but also associated with hormonal

problems, pregnancy, childbirth, the overuse of laxatives, and sitting on hard surfaces. *Hamamelis* is considered most effective for those type of haemorrhoids which, in appearance, resemble a bunch of grapes.

● **FIRST AID**
Hamamelis, also known as Virginian witch hazel, is valued as a herbal first aid remedy for its astringent properties.

● **BLEEDING**
This remedy is given to those with a susceptibility to haemorrhaging, such as women who suffer from heavy periods, or people who experience extreme nosebleeds.

Hepar sulph.

Eases respiratory problems ◆ Heals skin

infections ◆ Treats digestive disorders

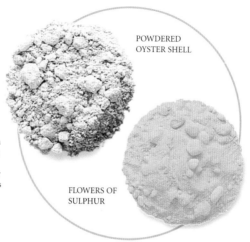

POWDERED
OYSTER SHELL

Hepar sulph. is a
form of calcium
sulphide using
powdered oyster
shell and flowers
of sulphur.

FLOWERS OF
SULPHUR

KEY ACTIONS

- REDUCES FEVER
- TREATS SWOLLEN
  GLANDS
- SOOTHES PAINFUL SKIN
- PROMOTES HEALING

KEY PREPARATIONS

- POWDER made from
  flowers of sulphur
  and powdered oyster
  shell. They are
  heated, dissolved in
  acid, and triturated
  with lactose sugar.

INDICATIONS

● **INFECTIONS**
Hepar sulph. is generally
used where there is an
infection, particularly in
the respiratory system or
the skin (such as styes,
boils, and cold sores). It is
particularly appropriate
for ailments that are
accompanied by swollen
glands, especially in the
neck or groin, or if there
is a high fever alternating
with chills.

● **COUGHS & COLDS**
Colds or influenza with
fever; sore throats with
swollen tonsils; dry,
hacking coughs; and
croup are treated with
Hepar sulph. It reduces
the risk of a secondary

infection, loosens phlegm,
and brings down fever.

● **SKIN CONDITIONS**
This remedy is prescribed
for skin that chaps or
roughens easily, or where
inflamed, sore acne is
present. It promotes
healing in skin where
eruptions are slow to heal
and prone to infection.

● **ABSCESSES & ULCERS**
Hepar sulph. is given to
treat abscesses or ulcers
that bleed easily and are
at risk of infection.

● **DIGESTION**
Use *Hepar sulph.* to treat
nausea, vomiting, and
chronic diarrhoea
accompanied by a
grumbling abdomen.

MERC. SOL.

Cures halitosis ◆ Treats oral and genital thrush

Relieves the symptoms of osteoarthritis

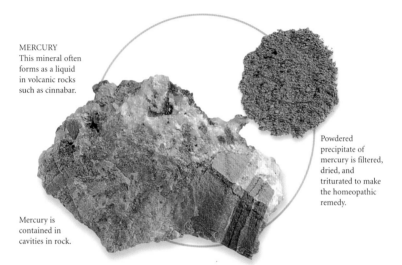

MERCURY
This mineral often forms as a liquid in volcanic rocks such as cinnabar.

Powdered precipitate of mercury is filtered, dried, and triturated to make the homeopathic remedy.

Mercury is contained in cavities in rock.

KEY ACTIONS

- FIGHTS INFECTION
- PAIN-RELIEVING
- SOOTHES MOUTH ULCERS AND ABSCESSES
- REDUCES FEVER

KEY PREPARATIONS

- POWDER made from mercury dissolved in nitric acid. This forms a grey powder precipitate which is filtered, dried, and triturated until soluble.

INDICATIONS

● **ARTHRITIS**
Merc. sol. is prescribed to relieve osteoarthritis.

● **HALITOSIS**
Halitosis (bad breath) can be caused by tooth decay, smoking, gingivitis, indigestion, tonsillitis, sinusitis, or fasting. Halitosis associated with tooth decay and gingivitis with bleeding gums, is treated with *Merc. sol.*

● **MOUTH & THROAT CONDITIONS**
Merc. sol. may be given for mouth ulcers; sore, raised, cream-coloured patches, usually indicative of oral thrush; abscesses; aching teeth caused by bleeding or infected gums; and sore throats.

● **THRUSH**
Merc. sol. treats thrush in men and women.

● **INFECTION**
Eye and ear infections can be alleviated by this remedy, as can colds, catarrh, and fever.

● **CAUTION**
Mercury, or "quicksilver", was used on its own as an aggressive treatment for syphilis and other diseases. It was given to Charles II and George Washington. Its use persisted to c. 1900 when it was stopped, in the West, its toxic effects deemed too dangerous.

HYOSCYAMUS

Alleviates the early symptoms of Parkinson's disease

Aids stroke victims ◆ Treats paranoia

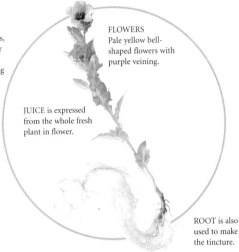

HENBANE
In the Middle Ages, the Latin name for henbane was *Dentaris*, signifying its use as a herbal remedy for toothache.

FLOWERS
Pale yellow bell-shaped flowers with purple veining.

JUICE is expressed from the whole fresh plant in flower.

ROOT is also used to make the tincture.

KEY ACTIONS

- ANTI-SPASMODIC
- SEDATIVE
- RELIEVES FEELINGS OF CONFUSION, JEALOUSY, AND PARANOIA

KEY PREPARATIONS

- OIL used in massage to relieve nerve pain and rheumatoid arthritis.
- TINCTURE made from the whole, fresh plant in flower, including the root. It is chopped finely, steeped in alcohol for 10 days, diluted, and succussed.

INDICATIONS

● **PARKINSON'S DISEASE**
The antispasmodic properties of *Hyoscyamus* (also known as henbane) are used by herbalists to relieve tremors and rigidity experienced during the early stages of Parkinson's disease.

● **STROKE**
Hyoscyamus is effective for treating a paralytic stroke that is associated with confused and inappropriate behaviour.

● **PARANOIA**
This remedy is given to sufferers of severe paranoia and jealousy, suspicious of being watched, deceived, or even poisoned. This may be exacerbated by PMS or emotional stress.

● **ANAESTHETIC**
The leaves are high in the sedative alkaloid hyoscine, used to make a conventional pre-operative anaesthetic.

● **CAUTION**
The leaves may cause skin irritation on contact. Taken internally, henbane is highly poisonous: it was the method by which Shakespeare had Hamlet's father murdered, and the infamous Dr Crippen used it to murder his unfortunate wife.

HYPERICUM

Prescribed for depression ◆ Prevents tetanus
Effective in treating phantom limb pain

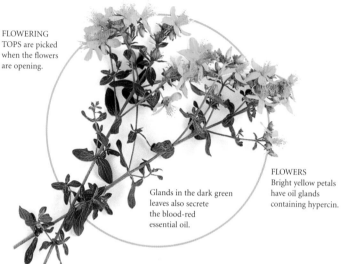

FLOWERING TOPS are picked when the flowers are opening.

FLOWERS
Bright yellow petals have oil glands containing hypercin.

Glands in the dark green leaves also secrete the blood-red essential oil.

KEY ACTIONS

- PAIN-RELIEVING
- CALMING
- CURES TOOTHACHE

KEY PREPARATIONS

- EXTRACT prescribed for depression.
- TINCTURE made from the whole, fresh plant. It is finely chopped and macerated in alcohol.

INDICATIONS

● **DEPRESSION**
Hypericum perf., also known as St. John's Wort, has been renowned since classical times. It is given to those who are shocked, frightened, or depressed. Those who benefit from it may be overexcited, nervous, continually drowsy, or forgetful. They may also experience a constant sensation of elevation or falling.

● **INJURIES**
Key physical symptoms associated with this remedy are injuries and wounds that feel more painful than they appear, with occurrences of extremely sharp pains,

perhaps in nerve-rich areas, such as the fingertips or the base of the spine. It may be used to relieve pain following operations, accidents, or puncture wounds.

● **ANIMAL BITES**
St. John's Wort may be administered to a patient who has been bitten by an animal; it is also given to help prevent tetanus.

● **PHANTOM LIMB PAIN**
The remedy is effective in treating pains experienced after amputation.

● **DENTAL CARE**
St. John's Wort is given to cure toothache. It is also used to relieve pain after dental surgery.

IGNATIA

Prescribed for acute grief

Relieves emotionalstress ◆ Treats insomnia

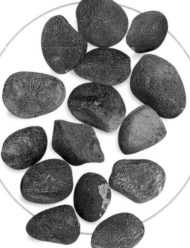

IGNATIA SEEDS
These seeds are very
bitter, due to the
poisonous
strychnine they
contain.

SEED PODS
Each seed pod
contains about
10 to 20 seeds.

The plant is native
to the East Indies,
China, and the
Phillipine Islands.

The seeds are separated
from the pulp and
powdered to make the
homeopathic remedy.

KEY ACTIONS

- CALMING
- AIDS WITH THE GRIEVING PROCESS
- PROMOTES GOOD DIGESTION
- TREATS MENSTRUAL PROBLEMS

KEY PREPARATIONS

- TINCTURE made from the dried seeds. They are powdered before being steeped in alcohol for at least five days. This is followed by filtration, dilution, and succussion.

INDICATIONS

● **GRIEF**
Ignatia is used to treat the initial impact of grief. It is particularly effective for women and is often given after a bereavement or the break-up of a relationship. Follow-up remedies may then be prescribed.

● **AMENORRHOEA**
Amenorrhoea is the absence of menstruation. Homeopaths may prescribe *Ignatia* when periods stop as a result of emotional stress.

● **STRESS**
The remedy is effective in treating illness that develops from emotional stress (*see above*). This includes: headaches; nervous tics and twitches; digestive disorders, such as nausea and vomiting; and a sore throat.

● **HICCUPS**
Hiccups associated with emotional stress are treated with *Ignatia*.

● **INSOMNIA**
Insomnia has several causes and effects. This remedy is prescribed for insomnia accompanied by a fear of never being able to fall asleep again.

● **CAUTION**
The seeds contain strychnine, a powerful poison that acts on the nervous system when ingested.

KALI. BICH.

Beneficial for the mucous membranes

Eases respiratory trouble ◆ Treats rheumatoid arthritis

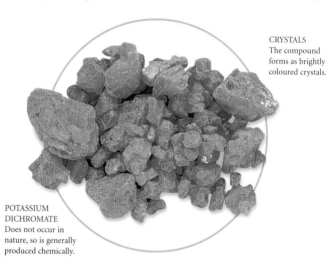

CRYSTALS
The compound forms as brightly coloured crystals.

POTASSIUM DICHROMATE
Does not occur in nature, so is generally produced chemically.

KEY ACTIONS

- ANTI-INFLAMMATORY
- PROMOTES SKIN HEALING
- FIGHTS INFECTION
- PAIN-RELIEVING

KEY PREPARATIONS

- TINCTURE made from crystals of potassium dichromate. These are finely ground (triturated) with lactose sugar until soluble in water. They are then filtered, diluted, and succussed.

INDICATIONS

● **ARTHRITIS**
Kali. bich. is prescribed for rheumatoid arthritis and other types of joint pain.

● **SINUSITIS**
Sinusitis occurs when the mucous membranes lining the sinuses become inflamed, due to allergy or infection. This remedy is effective for sinusitis with stringy catarrh.

● **GLUE EAR**
A condition resulting from overactivity of the mucous membrane lining the middle ear, or caused by allergy. A build up of sticky fluid leads to reduced hearing. If it is accompanied by thick,

stringy mucus, *Kali. bich.* may be prescribed.

● **BREATHING TROUBLE**
As *Kali. bich.* is considered beneficial for the mucous membranes (*see above*), it is given for respiratory-tract ailments, especially with excessive catarrh.

● **SKIN CONDITIONS**
The remedy is used to heal ulcers, acne, and other skin conditions accompanied by discharge or burning pain.

● **CAUTION**
Potassium dichromate, the compound used to make this remedy, is a powerful oxidizing agent and a highly caustic and corrosive poison.

KALI. CARB.

Prescribed for kidney disorders ◆ Treats whooping cough
and other chest infections ◆ Relieves insomnia

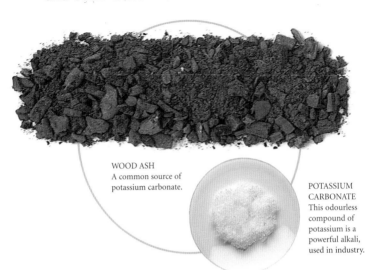

WOOD ASH
A common source of
potassium carbonate.

POTASSIUM
CARBONATE
This odourless
compound of
potassium is a
powerful alkali,
used in industry.

KEY ACTIONS

- PAIN-RELIEVING
- ANTI-INFLAMMATORY
- SOPORIFIC
- CALMING
- EASES OSTEOARTHRITIS

KEY PREPARATIONS

- LOTION used to heal
  skin complaints.
- TINCTURE made from
  potassium carbonate
  triturated by being
  ground repeatedly
  with lactose sugar
  until it is soluble in
  water. This solution is
  then diluted and
  succussed.

INDICATIONS

● **PAIN-RELIEF**
This remedy is associated
with pain in the joints,
back, or kidneys.

● **COUGHS & COLDS**
Dry, hacking, expectorant
coughs, whooping cough,
or wheezy coughs, may all
be treated with *Kali. carb.*

● **INSOMNIA**
Insomnia with difficulty
falling asleep, or getting to
sleep but waking again, is
treated with *Kali. carb.*

● **ASTHMA**
Kali. carb. is prescribed for
patients who regularly
suffer asthma attacks
between 2 a.m. and 4
a.m., causing exhaustion.

● **ARTHRITIS**
Kali. carb. is one of several
remedies indicated for
osteoarthritis.

● **PALPITATIONS**
It is given for palpitations
which are accompanied by
respiratory problems.

● **KIDNEY DISORDERS**
Kidney stones or other
diseases of the kidney are
treated with this remedy,
especially those with
shooting pains in the
small of the back. The
pains may be worse on the
left side.

● **CAUTION**
This is rarely prescribed
internally for medical
purposes, due to its
highly caustic nature.

KALI. MUR.

Key treatment for chronic catarrh ◆ Helps heal nasal
and aural problems ◆ Used in cancer treatment

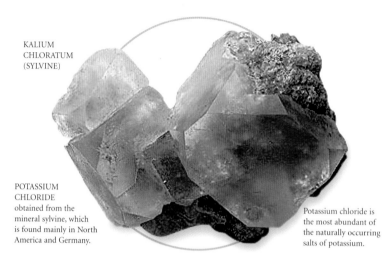

KALIUM
CHLORATUM
(SYLVINE)

POTASSIUM
CHLORIDE
obtained from the
mineral sylvine, which
is found mainly in North
America and Germany.

Potassium chloride is
the most abundant of
the naturally occurring
salts of potassium.

KEY ACTIONS

- ANTI-INFLAMMATORY
- RELIEVES CONGESTION
- PAIN-RELIEVING

KEY PREPARATIONS

- TISSUE SALTS made
  from powdered
  potassium chloride
  triturated with
  lactose sugar.

INDICATIONS

● **CANCER**
Kali. mur. is indicated in
the treatment for cancer
of the connective tissue
and of the throat.

● **NASAL PROBLEMS**
Congestion of the nose,
due to profuse, whitish
catarrh, and with the
presence of nosebleeds, is
treated with *Kali. mur.*

● **EARS**
The remedy is particularly
effective for the middle
ear, with accompanying
earache, pain behind the
ears, snapping noises,
blockage of the eustachian
tube (especially if
accompanied by catarrh),
and possible deafness.

● **TONSILLITIS**
Kali. mur. is an important
remedy for tonsillitis or
swollen throat glands. It is
also used for chronic sore
throats with catarrhal
crusts in the throat.

● **INFLAMMATION**
Kali. mur. is effective in
reducing inflammation; it
is most usually prescribed
to treat inflamed
membranes or joints.

● **EMOTIONS**
People who respond best
to *Kali. mur.* tend to be
optimistic and hard
working, but also tend to
alternate between
cheerfulness and sadness,
being sensitive to sadness
in others as well as in
themselves.

KREOSOTUM

Treats menstrual problems ◆ Key remedy for healing

mucous membranes ◆ Soothes candidiasis

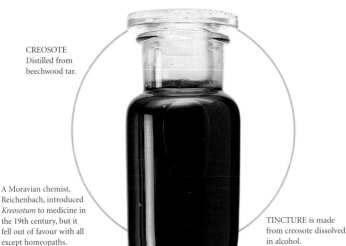

CREOSOTE
Distilled from
beechwood tar.

A Moravian chemist,
Reichenbach, introduced
Kreosotum to medicine in
the 19th century, but it
fell out of favour with all
except homeopaths.

TINCTURE is made
from creosote dissolved
in alcohol.

KEY ACTIONS

- ANTI-INFLAMMATORY
- SOOTHING
- TREATS CERTAIN
  EMOTIONAL PROBLEMS
- PROMOTES GOOD
  HEALTH IN WOMEN

KEY PREPARATIONS

- TINCTURE made from
  creosote dissolved in
  alcohol, diluted, and
  succussed.

INDICATIONS

● **MUCOUS MEMBRANES**
The classic symptom
picture associated with
Kreosotum is of mucous
membranes that become
inflamed, suppurate, and
break down and bleed,
particularly in the vagina,
cervix, and the uterus.

● **CANDIDIASIS**
Kreosotum is one of
several remedies that may
be prescribed to cure
candidiasis (thrush).

● **EMOTIONS & PHOBIAS**
People who respond best
to *Kreosotum* may be
temperamental, forgetful,
peevish, sensitive to
music, or restless at night.
A tendency to dwell on

the past, dreams of sexual
intercourse, and a fear of
being raped are typical.

● **DISCHARGE**
The remedy is given for
offensive-smelling
discharges from the
mucous membranes, that
burn the skin and cause
itching and swelling. It
may also help with
conditions where urine
burns the skin on contact.

● **MENSTRUATION**
It may be prescribed for
particular problems
associated with
menstruation, such as
bleeding between usual
cycles and heavy,
offensive-smelling
menstrual flow that burns
the skin on contact.

LACHESIS

Calms hot flushes ◆ Treats circulatory problems
Relieves spasms and tremors

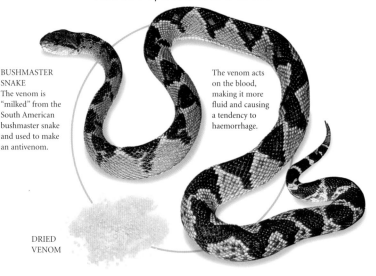

BUSHMASTER
SNAKE
The venom is
"milked" from the
South American
bushmaster snake
and used to make
an antivenom.

The venom acts
on the blood,
making it more
fluid and causing
a tendency to
haemorrhage.

DRIED
VENOM

KEY ACTIONS

- DEALS WITH LEFT-SIDED SYMPTOMS
- CALMING
- PAIN-RELIEVING
- ANTI-SPASMODIC

KEY PREPARATIONS

- TINCTURE made from venom "milked" from the bushmaster snake before being dissolved in alcohol. The mixture is then repeatedly diluted and succussed.

INDICATIONS

● **HOT FLUSHES**
Lachesis calms hot flushes that occur during the menopause, premenstrual syndrome, and certain nervous disorders.

● **ENERGY**
People who respond well to this remedy have fluctuating energy levels. When ill, symptoms may develop on the left side and develop or worsen during sleep.

● **CIRCULATION**
Poor circulation that turns the face, ears, and extremities blue or purple can be treated with *Lachesis*. It is prescribed for wounds that bleed

easily, and for engorged, bluish-purple varicose veins. It also treats cramping chest pains.

● **WOMEN'S HEALTH**
As well as hot flushes (*see above*), *Lachesis* is effective for painful menstruation, perhaps with fainting spells, palpitations, and hot sweats, and left-sided headaches or violent mood swings that occur premenstrually.

● **SPASMS & TREMORS**
Lachesis is given for muscle spasms, tremors, and weakness in the limbs, possibly linked to alcoholism, multiple sclerosis, fever, petit mal epilepsy, or brain damage after a stroke.

74

LEDUM

Eases painful joints and arthritic pain

Key first aid remedy ◆ Treats painful eye problems

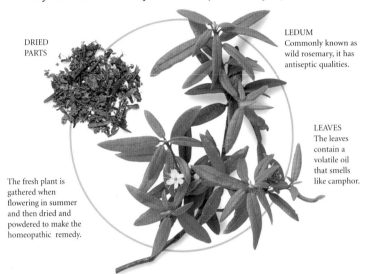

DRIED
PARTS

LEDUM
Commonly known as
wild rosemary, it has
antiseptic qualities.

LEAVES
The leaves
contain a
volatile oil
that smells
like camphor.

The fresh plant is
gathered when
flowering in summer
and then dried and
powdered to make the
homeopathic remedy.

KEY ACTIONS

- DISINFECTANT
- SLOWS BLEEDING
- ANTI-INFLAMMATORY

KEY PREPARATIONS

- TINCTURE made from
  the tips of the leafy
  shoots. They are
  collected as the plant
  comes into flower,
  then dried and
  steeped in alcohol.

INDICATIONS

● FIRST AID
This remedy is also
known as marsh tea and
wild rosemary. For years it
has been considered a key
first aid treatment for
cuts, grazes, puncture
wounds, insect stings, and
black eyes.

● PAINFUL JOINTS
Rheumatic pains that start
in the feet and move
upwards are relieved by
Ledum, as are stiff, painful
joints that feel hot inside
despite being cold to the
touch. For osteoarthritis
sufferers, the remedy is
given for joints that feel
cold, are swollen, and
make cracking noises on
moving. If a joint

complaint is relieved by
cold compresses, it will
respond well to *Ledum*.

● EYE CONDITIONS
As well as treating black
eyes (*see above*), especially
those slow to heal, *Ledum*
treats other eye injuries
including stemming
bleeding into the eye
chamber after an
iridectomy (removal
of part of the iris).

● INFECTION
Ledum prevents infection
in open wounds, such as
severe wounds with
bruised, puffy, purplish
skin and stinging pains.
Its disinfectant properties
led to its traditional use in
Scandinavia: to eliminate
body lice.

LILIUM

Prescribed for angina and other heart disorders

Used for women's health problems ◆ Treats depression

TIGER LILY
The bright-orange flowers of this lily appear in late summer and early autumn.

The fresh plant in flower is used to make the remedy.

PETALS
Bright petals curl up to reveal distinctive spots.

This native to China and Japan is now grown worldwide.

KEY ACTIONS

- TREATS URINARY DISORDERS
- CALMING
- PAIN-RELIEVING
- EMOTIONALLY UPLIFTING

KEY PREPARATIONS

- TINCTURE made from the stalk, leaves, and flowers of the fresh plant. They are chopped finely and soaked in alcohol for at least 10 days. The mixture is then filtered, diluted, and succussed.

INDICATIONS

● **URINARY DISORDERS**
Cystitis (usually in women) with burning, stinging pain during and after urination is treated with this remedy. It helps to reduce the patient's constant need to pass urine when only a small amount is being passed at any one time.

● **WOMEN'S HEALTH**
Disorders of the female reproductive system, such as uterine prolapse, vulval itching, and a bearing-down pain in the pelvis, may be treated with *Lilium*. Fibroids may also be treated with the remedy, and it may be recommended for swollen ovaries or painful menstruation.

● **DEPRESSION**
A sense of despair and a need for religious salvation is characteristic in people who need *Lilium*. They may have a fear of developing an incurable disease and look for a reason to grieve.

● **ANGINA**
Lilium is prescribed when the chest feels as though it is being gripped in a vice, and there are palpitations and pain in the right arm. It is also given for other heart disorders, such as rapid or irregular pulse, poor circulation, or palpitations that occur during pregnancy.

LYCOPODIUM

Treats urogenitary and prostate disorders

Eases anxiety ◆ Alleviates digestive problems

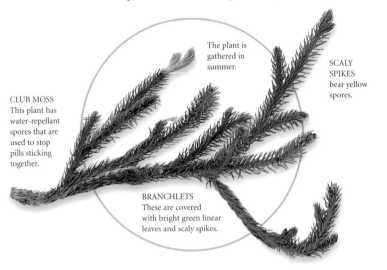

The plant is gathered in summer.

SCALY SPIKES bear yellow spores.

CLUB MOSS This plant has water-repellant spores that are used to stop pills sticking together.

BRANCHLETS These are covered with bright green linear leaves and scaly spikes.

KEY ACTIONS

- ANTIBACTERIAL
- SEDATIVE
- FIGHTS INFECTION
- CALMING

KEY PREPARATIONS

- TINCTURE made from the spikes of Lycopodium. They are cut in summer and their spores are collected. These are then steeped in alcohol for at least five days, before being filtered, diluted, and succussed.

INDICATIONS

● **PROSTATE PROBLEMS**
Lycopodium is one of several homeopathic remedies recommended for prostate disorders. It is prescribed when the prostate has become enlarged. It is also given to treat urine with a sandy sediment due to kidney stones, and for genital herpes. It was used in the 17th century to ease urine retention.

● **ANXIETY**
Traditionally used for its sedative action, this remedy is prescribed to those who suffer from insomnia, talking and laughing while asleep, night fears, and apprehension upon waking. Anticipatory anxiety, such as fear of public speaking, exams, or performing onstage, all of which often lead to digestive disorders, are treated with *Lycopodium.*

● **DIGESTIVE DISORDER**
This remedy is given for indigestion, such as that caused by anticipatory anxiety (*see above*); nausea; vomiting; constipation; and bleeding haemorrhoids.

● **CHEST INFECTIONS**
Dry, sore, tickling coughs; burning chest pains; and fast, laboured breathing can be eased with *Lycopodium*; as can sore throats and severe catarrh.

MAG. PHOS.

Treats neuralgia ◆ Eases abdominal pains and other cramps

Relieves headaches, toothache, and earache

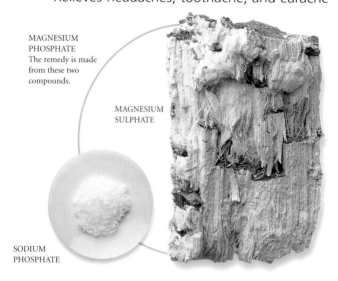

MAGNESIUM
PHOSPHATE
The remedy is made
from these two
compounds.

MAGNESIUM
SULPHATE

SODIUM
PHOSPHATE

KEY ACTIONS

- PAIN-RELIEVING
- ANTI-SPASMODIC
- DEALS CHIEFLY WITH
  RIGHT-SIDED PAIN
- SOOTHES MENSTRUAL
  CRAMPS
- RELIEVES IRRITABLE
  BOWEL SYNDROME

KEY PREPARATIONS

- TISSUE SALTS made
  from magnesium
  sulphate and sodium
  phosphate mixed in
  water and left to
  crystallize. The
  resulting crystals are
  then triturated with
  lactose sugar.

INDICATIONS

● **MENSTRUAL CRAMPS**
Taken for sudden
cramping, shooting pains
in the lower abdomen
during menstruation. Also
given for non-menstrual
abdominal cramps, such
as those associated with
Irritable Bowel Syndrome.

● **EARACHE**
The remedy relieves pains
in the ear that are
spasmodic and shooting,
especially following
exposure to cold wind.

● **TOOTHACHE**
Dull, throbbing pain, or
sharp twinges of pain,
especially common in
teething infants, can be
treated with *Mag. phos.*

● **NEURALGIA**
Mag. phos. is prescribed
for sharp, radiating,
cramping pains that
appear and disappear
rapidly anywhere in the
body. It relieves muscles
that are stiff, numb, and
awkward, especially after
exertion.

● **HEADACHE**
Given for spasmodic,
shooting pains on the
right side, or back of the
neck; pains that spread
over the head and settle
around the right eye.

● **CRAMPS**
Treats sudden onset of
cramps in the fingers,
arms, wrists, and hands,
common in musicians
and writers.

NAT. MUR.

Used for women's health disorders ◆ Promotes good
digestion ◆ Relieves migraines and headaches

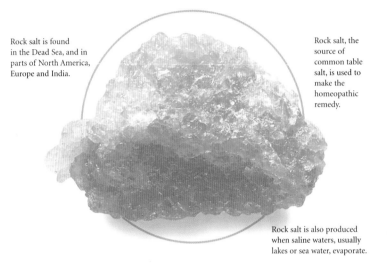

Rock salt is found
in the Dead Sea, and in
parts of North America,
Europe and India.

Rock salt, the
source of
common table
salt, is used to
make the
homeopathic
remedy.

Rock salt is also produced
when saline waters, usually
lakes or sea water, evaporate.

KEY ACTIONS

- HEALS MOUTH ULCERS,
  ABSCESSES AND
  GINGIVITIS
- EASES MENSTRUAL
  PROBLEMS
- SOOTHES SKIN
  CONDITIONS

KEY PREPARATIONS

- POWDER made from
  rock salt dissolved in
  boiling water,
  filtered, and
  evaporated to make
  pure sodium
  chloride. This is then
  triturated with
  lactose sugar.
  Historically, salt had
  economic value, but
  has had limited
  medicinal uses
  outside homeopathy.

INDICATIONS

● **HEADACHES**
The remedy relieves
hammering, bursting
headaches, and migraines,
that occur above the eyes.
It also treats those
headaches and migraines
accompanied by vision
distortion, such as
zigzag lines.

● **DIGESTION**
Nat. mur. is prescribed for
constipation where the
stools are dry and hard,
causing colicky pains with
nausea, backache, and
possible anal bleeding.

● **WOMEN'S HEALTH**
Used to cure fatigue, water
retention, and severe
headaches occurring
around menstruation.
Also given to treat white
vaginal discharge, usually
due to thrush. Has been
effective in treating
vaginismus, where painful
spasms occur during
intercourse, and for
patients whose periods
have stopped due to grief
or shock.

● **SKIN CONDITIONS**
Greasy skin and hair,
dandruff, warts, boils,
psoriasis, urticaria (hives),
hangnails, and facial cold
sores may be helped by
the remedy.

● **MOUTH & THROAT**
Nat. mur. heals mouth
ulcers, dental abscesses,
gingivitis (bleeding
gums), and cracked lips.

NAT. SULPH.

Eases liver problems ◆ Associated with head symptoms

Key remedy for asthma

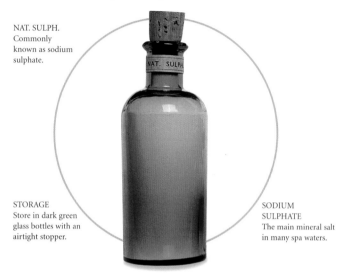

NAT. SULPH.
Commonly known as sodium sulphate.

STORAGE
Store in dark green glass bottles with an airtight stopper.

SODIUM SULPHATE
The main mineral salt in many spa waters.

KEY ACTIONS

- PROMOTES GOOD DIGESTION
- TREATS DEPRESSION
- SOOTHES HEADACHES
- USED FOR HEPATITIS
- EASES GALLSTONES

KEY PREPARATIONS

- TISSUE SALTS made from sodium sulphate triturated with lactose sugar.

INDICATIONS

● **HEADACHES**
Nat. sulph. has an affinity with head symptoms, such as headaches due to injury, or those accompanied by increased salivation or strong intolerance to light.

● **DEPRESSION**
The remedy is prescribed for severe or suicidal depression, and for profound mental changes, possibly with suicidal thoughts, following a head injury.

● **EMOTIONS**
Nat. sulph. is best suited to people who are serious, reserved, responsible, and focused on work, yet paradoxically highly sensitive; music may move them to tears. They may feel isolated from intimate, committed relationships, perhaps after losing a partner.

● **ASTHMA**
This is a major remedy for asthma brought on by damp conditions.

● **LIVER PROBLEMS**
Problems with the liver, the digestive system, gallbladder, pancreas, and spleen may be treated with *Nat. sulph.* Liver conditions treated by the remedy include hepatitis and gallstones with bitter belching, colicky abdominal pains, and jaundice.

OPIUM

Alleviates insomnia ◆ Helps with post-stroke treatment

Used to treat shock

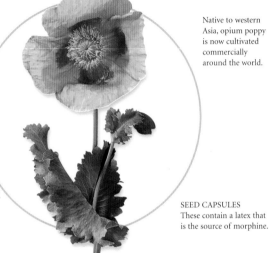

OPIUM POPPY
Flowers appear in late summer and early autumn.

Native to western Asia, opium poppy is now cultivated commercially around the world.

The plant has dull green leaves and thick stems.

SEED CAPSULES
These contain a latex that is the source of morphine.

KEY ACTIONS

- RELIEVES CONSTIPATION
- TREATS DELIRIUM TREMENS
- HELPS WITH NARCOLEPSY
- AIDS ALCOHOL WITHDRAWAL

KEY PREPARATIONS

- MORPHINE used in conventional medicine.
- TINCTURE made from the sap of the unripe green seed pods, dried, dissolved in alcohol, and succussed.

INDICATIONS

● **DELIRIUM TREMENS**
Extreme apathy or hypersensitivity, tremors, or convulsions resulting from delirium tremens are treated with *Opium*. It is also prescribed to aid with alcohol withdrawal.

● **SHOCK & INJURY**
Emotional responses to shock, grief, or injury can be treated with *Opium*, as can physical responses, such as convulsions.

● **INSOMNIA**
Opium has been used as a sedative and analgesic since antiquity. It was dedicated by the Greeks and Romans to the gods of night, death, and dreams. Insomnia, an inability to sleep despite fatigue, and brief bouts of irresistible drowsiness can be treated with *Opium*. It is also indicated for the treatment of narcolepsy.

● **CONSTIPATION**
Newborn babies may be given *Opium* to relieve constipation after the shock of birth. Children and adults are also treated with the remedy.

● **POST-STROKE CARE**
The remedy treats paralysis of the limbs with dullness and stupor resembling that experienced after shock, possibly with blackouts. It is also used for resultant brain injuries.

PHOSPHORUS

Stems heavy bleeding ◆ Helps with poor circulation

Treats respiratory problems

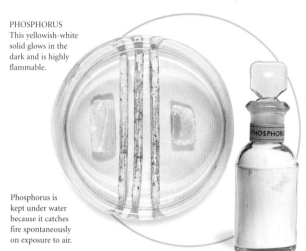

PHOSPHORUS
This yellowish-white solid glows in the dark and is highly flammable.

PHOSPHORUS REMEDY

Phosphorus is kept under water because it catches fire spontaneously on exposure to air.

Profuse bleeding from the gums is one of the conditions helped by this remedy.

KEY ACTIONS

- CALMING
- TREATS ASTHMA, BRONCHITIS, AND PNEUMONIA
- IMPROVES CIRCULATION
- PROMOTES GOOD DIGESTION

KEY PREPARATIONS

- TINCTURE made from white phosphorus. This waxy substance is insoluble in water, so it is dissolved in alcohol, filtered, then repeatedly diluted and succussed.

INDICATIONS

● **DIGESTIVE PROBLEMS**
Phosphorus is given for digestive disorders where the stools are streaked with blood. It may be prescribed for stomach ulcers, gastroenteritis, food poisoning, and stomach trouble caused by stress.

● **BLEEDING**
Profuse bleeding, from the nose, gums, and stomach lining, is treated with *Phosphorus*. It is also given for heavy menstrual flow.

● **POOR CIRCULATION**
Given to reduce the effects of poor circulation, including: erratic blood flow causing hot flushes;

palpitations; and fainting, characterized by a weak pulse. Treats extremities that feel burning hot yet are cold to the touch.

● **RESPIRATORY ILLNESS**
The remedy is used for respiratory problems linked to anxiety and is associated with chest tightness due to asthma, bronchitis, or pneumonia. Symptoms treated may include phlegm streaked with dark-red blood, a sore throat, dry tickly cough, and possible retching or vomiting.

● **CAUTION**
Overexposure to the white form of the element can be deadly, since it is highly toxic.

PHYTOLACCA

Eases breast problems ◆ Heals psoriasis

Treats glandular fever and other glandular disorders

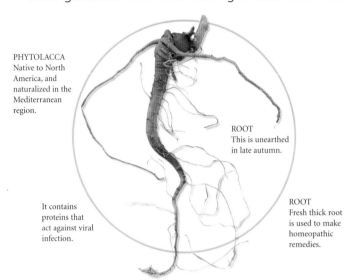

PHYTOLACCA
Native to North America, and naturalized in the Mediterranean region.

ROOT
This is unearthed in late autumn.

It contains proteins that act against viral infection.

ROOT
Fresh thick root is used to make homeopathic remedies.

KEY ACTIONS

- ANTI-INFLAMMATORY
- PAIN-RELIEVING
- GIVEN FOR MUMPS
- EASES DIFFICULT BREATHING

KEY PREPARATIONS

- TINCTURE made from the fresh root, unearthed during the autumn. It is finely chopped and macerated in alcohol.

INDICATIONS

● **BREAST PROBLEMS**
Prescribed to treat cysts that are tender before and during menstruation. It is also given for breast ulcers and sometimes for breast cancer. *Phytolacca* treats mastitis with hardness, burning, and pain in the breasts that radiates through the whole body on breast-feeding.

● **PSORIASIS**
Phytolacca is prescribed to sufferers of psoriasis when there are lesions with a purple coloration present.

● **GLANDS**
This remedy has a strong affinity with the glands and is used to treat glandular fever. It is given for hard, inflamed neck glands, where pain in the throat is present upon swallowing. Inflamed parotid glands, for example during mumps, may be helped by the remedy. Also given for inflamed, painful tonsils, which may appear dark red in colour.

● **BREATHING**
When breathing feels difficult, restricted, and oppressed, with a sense of suffocation and emptiness in the chest, *Phytolacca* may be prescribed.

● **CAUTION**
This plant is highly potent and toxic if taken in excess.

PULSATILLA

Heals eye infections ◆ Useful remedy for gynaecological problems ◆ Relieves sinusitis

FLOWERING PLANT
The whole fresh flowering plant is pulped and the juice expressed to make the homeopathic remedy.

BELL-SHAPED FLOWERS

FLOWERS
The plant is distinguished from other *Pulsatilla* species by its smaller, purplish black flowerheads.

FEATHERY LEAVES

ROOTS
These are pulped with the rest of the plant to express the juice.

KEY ACTIONS

- REDUCES FEVER
- PROMOTES GOOD DIGESTION
- EASES COUGHS AND COLDS
- TREATS INFLUENZA
- HELPS WITH PRE-MENSTRUAL SYNDROME

KEY PREPARATIONS

- TINCTURE made from the fresh flowering plant, including the root. It is chopped and macerated in alcohol, before being diluted and succussed.

INDICATIONS

● **EYE INFECTIONS**
Roman legend says this plant sprang from the tears of Venus, and was hence used for weepiness. *Pulsatilla* may help itchy eyes and conjunctivitis. In the 1st century AD, Dioscorides, the Greek physician, prescribed it for eye problems.

● **WOMEN'S HEALTH**
Given for short, variable, late, or absent periods, and for severe menstrual pain. PMS may also respond to the remedy and it is sometimes given to pregnant women, if the symptom picture fits. It can also be used to act on the uterine muscles and help turn a breech baby during labour.

● **SINUSITIS**
Pulsatilla is given when the sinuses are tender to the touch, with sharp pains beginning on the right side of the face, but tending to move around.

● **COUGHS & COLDS**
Treats wet, spasmodic coughing, with shortness of breath, worse for lying on the left side. *Pulsatilla* may also be prescribed for influenza with fever.

● **DIGESTIVE PROBLEMS**
Used for varied problems, including vomiting, nausea, indigestion, diarrhoea, and painful, itchy haemorrhoids.

RHUS TOX.

Eases musculo-skeletal pain ◆ Heals infected skin
Soothes other painful skin complaints

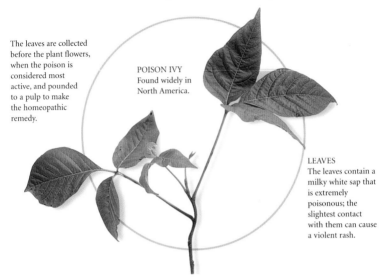

The leaves are collected before the plant flowers, when the poison is considered most active, and pounded to a pulp to make the homeopathic remedy.

POISON IVY
Found widely in North America.

LEAVES
The leaves contain a milky white sap that is extremely poisonous; the slightest contact with them can cause a violent rash.

KEY ACTIONS

- ANTI-INFLAMMATORY
- FIGHTS INFECTIONS
- EASES ARTHRITIC PAIN
- TREATS ECZEMA AND OTHER SKIN PROBLEMS

KEY PREPARATIONS

- TINCTURE made from the fresh leaves, gathered at sunset just before the plant comes into flower. These are macerated in alcohol.

INDICATIONS

● **JOINTS**
Musculo-skeletal problems are associated with *Rhus tox.* and this remedy has become associated specifically with the joints. It is used to ease acute arthritis – both osteo- and rheumatoid – as well as sciatica, restless legs, cramps, strains, and sprains.

● **SKIN INFECTIONS**
As well as joint problems (*see above*), *Rhus tox.* is associated primarily with infection of the skin. It is effective for eczema and for conditions such as Rosacea, where boils start to form. Infected eczema may start to ooze. The condition may be an allergic reaction, but the cause is often unknown. Childhood eczema usually clears up by puberty.

● **SKIN CONDITIONS**
Native Americans used this plant to treat skin eruptions and nervous paralysis. It may be helpful for skin eruptions with blisters, followed by burning, red, swollen skin that tends to scale and flake off. The remedy is given to treat chicken pox, shingles, herpes, and nappy rash.

● **CAUTION**
Contact with the plant's leaves produces redness, swelling, and blistering.

RUTA

Prescribed for eyestrain ◆ Eases muscular problems

Alleviates painful joints

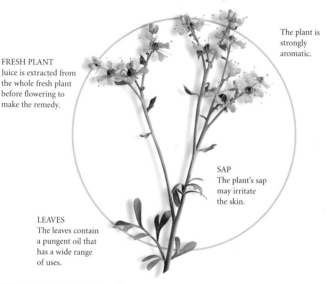

The plant is strongly aromatic.

FRESH PLANT
Juice is extracted from the whole fresh plant before flowering to make the remedy.

SAP
The plant's sap may irritate the skin.

LEAVES
The leaves contain a pungent oil that has a wide range of uses.

KEY ACTIONS

- CALMING
- PAIN-RELIEVING
- HEALS STRAINED MUSCLES
- RELIEVES STIFFNESS IN MUSCLES AND JOINTS

KEY PREPARATIONS

- TINCTURE made from the aerial parts, gathered as the plant is beginning to flower. They are finely chopped and steeped in alcohol.

INDICATIONS

● **MENSTRUATION**
Ruta (also known as "Rue" or "herb-of-grace") has been prescribed herbally since the times of ancient Egypt and Greece to induce abortion and stimulate menstruation. The remedy may be given for menstrual problems.

● **MUSCLE PROBLEMS**
The classic symptom picture for *Ruta* is of connective tissue problems with marked stiffness and pain in the muscles and tendons, often due to sprains, overuse of the muscles, or injury. The pain is typically sore, bruised, aching, and accompanied

by restlessness. The remedy is prescribed for repetitive strain injury.

● **EYE TREATMENTS**
Ruta is used to treat eyestrain (when the muscles have become weak), where burning pain is experienced. In ancient times the plant was used medicinally to strengthen eye sight.

● **JOINT PROBLEMS**
Used to treat chronic arthritis, a stiff, sore lower back, and sciatica.

● **EMOTIONS**
Those who respond best to the *Ruta* remedy are prone to feelings of anxiety and panic and tend to be weepy.

SEPIA

Treats women's health problems ◆ Soothes painful

skin conditions ◆ Improves circulation

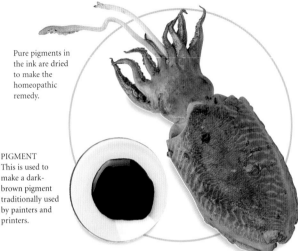

Pure pigments in
the ink are dried
to make the
homeopathic
remedy.

This soft mollusc
is related to the
octopus and
squid. It squirts
brownish-black
ink for protection.

PIGMENT
This is used to
make a dark-
brown pigment
traditionally used
by painters and
printers.

KEY ACTIONS

- PAIN-RELIEVING
- SOOTHING
- CORRECTS HORMONAL
  IMBALANCE
- AIDS DIGESTION

KEY PREPARATIONS

- POWDER made from
  cuttlefish ink dried
  to a crystalline form
  and then triturated
  with lactose sugar.

INDICATIONS

● **WOMEN'S HEALTH**
Sepia, or cuttlefish ink, is
predominantly prescribed
to treat women's health
problems, including
hormone imbalances,
especially those that occur
before or during
menstruation, or
throughout menopause.
It is also prescribed for
some pregnancy-related
ailments and can be used
to treat thrush.

● **DIGESTIVE PROBLEMS**
Helps relieve indigestion,
flatulence, vomiting,
nausea, and constipation.

● **SKIN CONDITIONS**
The remedy is prescribed
for itchy, or discoloured

skin and a condition
known as chloasma in
which a yellow-brown
"saddle" appears across
the nose and cheeks,
especially during
pregnancy.

● **CIRCULATION**
The remedy is given for
palpitations, varicose
veins, and hot and cold
flushes.

● **PAIN RELIEF**
Treats headaches that are
prevalent on the left side,
possibly with dizziness
and nausea. Also relieves
painful catarrh, and signs
of emotional and physical
exhaustion, especially
those accompanied by an
aching back and sides and
muscles that feel weak.

SILICA

Strengthens bones, teeth, hair, and nails

Promotes skin healing ◆ Treats food intolerances

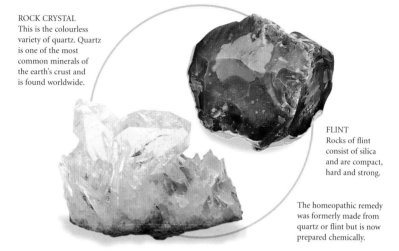

ROCK CRYSTAL
This is the colourless variety of quartz. Quartz is one of the most common minerals of the earth's crust and is found worldwide.

FLINT
Rocks of flint consist of silica and are compact, hard and strong.

The homeopathic remedy was formerly made from quartz or flint but is now prepared chemically.

KEY ACTIONS

- HEALING
- STRENGTHENING
- SOOTHING
- PAIN-RELIEVING
- FIGHTS INFECTION
- REMOVES FOREIGN BODIES FROM THE SKIN

KEY PREPARATIONS

- TINCTURE made by triturating silicon dioxide, grinding the sand repeatedly with lactose sugar until it becomes soluble in water, then diluting and succussing it.

INDICATIONS

● **BONES & TEETH**
Silica promotes healing in brittle bones, and is given for curvature of the spine. It is used for slow-healing problems and to improve children's health, such as fontanelles that close slowly. It is also given for slow eruption of teeth and to ease wisdom teething.

● **SKIN, HAIR, & NAILS**
The remedy heals defects due to poor absorption of minerals in the diet. It heals brittle, distorted, infected nails and ingrown toenails. It is used to encourages healing in wounds that suppurate and heal slowly, abscesses, itchy scars, and acne.

● **REMOVING SPLINTERS**
Silica has the unusual feature of reputedly being able to help expel foreign bodies such as splinters from the skin.

● **HEADACHES**
Severe pain starting at the back of the head and extending over to the forehead, with dizziness and visual disturbances, is treated with *Silica*.

● **DIGESTIVE PROBLEMS**
Prescribed for a weak digestive system, with food intolerances.

● **COUGHS & COLDS**
Silica is used for persistent or recurrent coughs, colds, and infections of the ear, nose, and throat.

DULCAMARA

Eases painful joints ◆ Treats hay fever and asthma

Relieves head and facial pain

This plant has a long history of use as an anti-inflammatory and a liver tonic. Stem extracts have been used for warts and eczema.

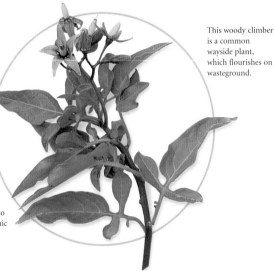

This woody climber is a common wayside plant, which flourishes on wasteground.

LEAVES
Young green shoots and leaves of the fresh plant are used to make the homeopathic remedy.

KEY ACTIONS

- PAIN-RELIEVING
- ANTI-INFLAMMATORY
- SOOTHING
- EASES CONGESTION

KEY PREPARATIONS

- TINCTURE made from fresh green leaves and stems, which are picked just before the plant flowers. They are finely chopped and macerated in alcohol.

INDICATIONS

● **JOINT PAIN**
The remedy is typically given to people who are sensitive to cold and damp; it relieves joint pain and stiffness, aggravated by damp.

● **DIARRHOEA**
Given for diarrhoea that may be accompanied by blood. Also prescribed for diarrhoea caused by teething in babies.

● **SKIN CONDITIONS**
Dulcamara is given to promote healing of the skin; the remedy is effective for thickening of the epidermis. It treats eczema, urticaria (hives), warts, and ringworm.

● **COUGHS & COLDS**
Treats pneumonia, bronchitis, coughs and colds, as well as associated sore throats, stiffness in the neck, or pain in the back or limbs.

● **HAY FEVER & ASTHMA**
Eases nasal congestion, constricted breathing, and watery eyes.

● **HEAD & FACIAL PAIN**
Relieves neuralgic pain, including that caused by Bell's palsy or sinusitis.

● **CAUTION**
Dulcamara (bittersweet) is highly toxic and therefore used only by trained herbalists. The leaves and unripe berries are the most toxic part.

SPIGELIA

Treats problems of the nervous system ◆ Eases arthritis

Relieves angina and other heart conditions

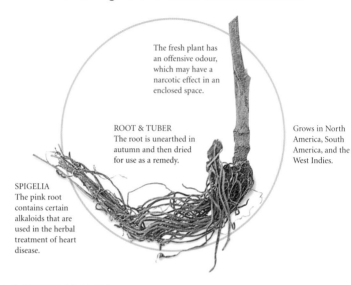

The fresh plant has an offensive odour, which may have a narcotic effect in an enclosed space.

ROOT & TUBER
The root is unearthed in autumn and then dried for use as a remedy.

Grows in North America, South America, and the West Indies.

SPIGELIA
The pink root contains certain alkaloids that are used in the herbal treatment of heart disease.

KEY ACTIONS

- PAIN-RELIEVING
- CALMS PALPITATIONS
- USED TO TREAT PROBLEMS PRIMARILY ON THE LEFT SIDE OF THE BODY

KEY PREPARATIONS

- TINCTURE made from the dried aerial parts which are macerated in alcohol.
- ROOT The pink part of which is used in the herbal treatment of heart disease.

INDICATIONS

● NERVOUS SYSTEM
As well as heart conditions (*see below*), *Spigelia* is given chiefly for problems with the nervous system, especially if symptoms primarily affect the left side of the body, and if there are intense, violent pains.

● PAIN RELIEF
Given for headaches, migraines, sinus infections, and neuralgic and rheumatic pain.

● HEART CONDITIONS
The pink root contains alkaloids used in herbal heart treatments. The remedy is also used for problems associated with the heart. *Spigelia* may be given for frequent palpitations that are violent, visible, and audible; for heart murmurs or valve disorders; and for rheumatic heart disease.

● ANGINA
Spigelia is also used for angina with constricting chest pains that extend down one or both arms, into the chest, and up to the throat.

● ARTHRITIS
Spigelia is prescribed to sufferers of rheumatoid arthritis, to alleviate tearing pains near the joints, that feel as though a knife were scraping along the bones.

ANTIMONIUM CRUD.

Heals skin and nail conditions

Treats digestive problems ◆ Relieves gout

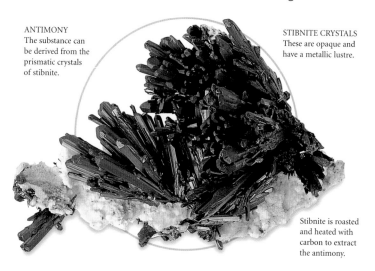

ANTIMONY
The substance can be derived from the prismatic crystals of stibnite.

STIBNITE CRYSTALS
These are opaque and have a metallic lustre.

Stibnite is roasted and heated with carbon to extract the antimony.

KEY ACTIONS

- FIGHTS INFECTION
- ANTI-INFLAMMATORY
- PAIN-RELIEVING
- REDUCES FEVER

KEY PREPARATIONS

- TINCTURE made from stibnite which is roasted and heated with carbon to extract the antimony. It is then triturated with lactose sugar, diluted, and succussed.

INDICATIONS

● **BEAUTY TREATMENT**
Antimony occurs naturally in crystalline form as stibnite, which was used as kohl, by women in ancient Rome and the Middle East.

● **SKIN INFECTIONS**
A rash on the trunk, arms, and legs, or itchy rashes that become worse when hot, may be treated with *Antimonium crud.*

● **DIGESTIVE PROBLEMS**
Given for indigestion with belching, nausea, and vomiting of bile, especially caused by overindulgence or pregnancy. It is given to babies who vomit breast milk and will not suckle, or to their mothers. It is also used for diarrhoea and constipation.

● **SKIN & NAILS**
Treats callouses, warts, and corns that may form on the hands, under the fingernails, on the soles of the feet, and on the tips of the toes. Also used to treat nails that split repeatedly.

● **GOUT**
Inflammation and redness in affected joints is treated with *Antimonium crud.* It also alleviates mild fevers and tense, jumpy muscles.

● **TOOTHACHE**
Relieves persistent, gnawing toothache, usually caused by decaying teeth.

91

NUX VOMICA

Alleviates insomnia ◆ May be used safely

during pregnancy ◆ Relieves digestive disorders

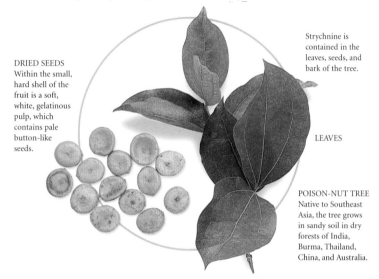

DRIED SEEDS
Within the small, hard shell of the fruit is a soft, white, gelatinous pulp, which contains pale button-like seeds.

Strychnine is contained in the leaves, seeds, and bark of the tree.

LEAVES

POISON-NUT TREE
Native to Southeast Asia, the tree grows in sandy soil in dry forests of India, Burma, Thailand, China, and Australia.

KEY ACTIONS

- RELIEVES CRAMPS
- CALMS IRRITABILITY
- REDUCES FEVER
- EFFECTIVE FOR TREATMENT OF PREMENSTRUAL SYNDROME

KEY PREPARATIONS

- BARK Used by Indian herbalists to treat cholera and, in Nepal, prescribed for menstrual problems, rabies, and paralysis.
- TINCTURE made from the dried, ripe seeds which are steeped in alcohol for at least five days, before being filtered, diluted, and succussed.

INDICATIONS

● **DIGESTIVE PROBLEMS**
Given for indigestion; vomiting with painful retching; diarrhoea with abdominal cramps; and nausea with colicky pain.

● **INSOMNIA**
Insomnia with hangover-like symptoms, or disrupted sleep, with great irascibility, is treated with *Nux vomica*.

● **COLDS & INFLUENZA**
Treats symptoms such as catarrh; dry, tickly coughs; headaches; shivery fever; and sensitive eyes.

● **WOMEN'S HEALTH**
The remedy is given for cystitis with spasmodic pain in the bladder and a frequent desire to urinate; early, irregular, or heavy menstruation; faintness during menstruation; and premenstrual syndrome with a violent temper.

● **PREGNANCY**
Nux vomica may be used during pregnancy to help ease fatigue, frequent urination, numbness in the arms, leg cramps, constipation, and morning sickness.

● **CAUTION**
In large doses, the strychnine present in this plant induces intense spasms of the diaphragm, causing respiration to cease and death by suffocation.

SULPHUR

Prescribed for impotence in men ◆ Soothes painful skin conditions ◆ Treats gynaecological problems

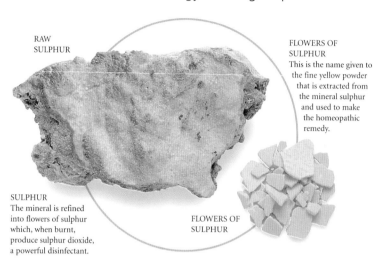

RAW
SULPHUR

FLOWERS OF
SULPHUR
This is the name given to
the fine yellow powder
that is extracted from
the mineral sulphur
and used to make
the homeopathic
remedy.

SULPHUR
The mineral is refined
into flowers of sulphur
which, when burnt,
produce sulphur dioxide,
a powerful disinfectant.

FLOWERS OF
SULPHUR

KEY ACTIONS

- ANTISEPTIC
- ANTI-INFLAMMATORY
- PROMOTES GOOD DIGESTION
- EASES BREATHING PROBLEMS

KEY PREPARATIONS

- TINCTURE made from chemically purified sulphur. It is triturated by grinding it into a fine powder that is soluble in water and alcohol.

INDICATIONS

● **VITALITY**
Sulphur is prescribed for a broader range of ailments than any other remedy. It is given to boost vitality and clear up lingering illnesses.

● **SKIN CONDITIONS**
Long used in Chinese and Western medicine for skin problems. It is used for nappy rash, cradle cap, acne, psoriasis, eczema, ringworm, and scabies.

● **WOMEN'S HEALTH**
Given for painful or irregular menstruation; relieves headaches, irritability, and insomnia associated with PMS; and hot flushes, dizziness, and sweats associated with the menopause. It also treats thrush and cystitis.

● **MEN'S HEALTH**
Sulphur is prescribed for impotence or erectile failure accompanied by sharp pains in the penis and itching in the tip of the penis. Penis or prostate inflammation may also be helped.

● **DIGESTIVE PROBLEMS**
The remedy relieves bloating, belching, indigestion, flatulence, vomiting, and diarrhoea.

● **BREATHING TROUBLE**
Helps treat coughs and colds, preventing them from developing into bronchitis or pneumonia.

TARENTULA

Used by multiple sclerosis sufferers ◆ Prescribed for
gynaecological problems ◆ Treats heart problems

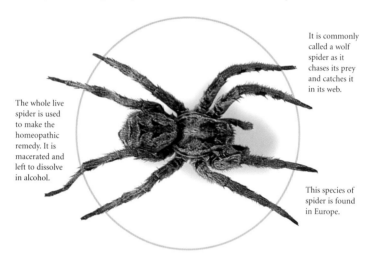

It is commonly called a wolf spider as it chases its prey and catches it in its web.

The whole live spider is used to make the homeopathic remedy. It is macerated and left to dissolve in alcohol.

This species of spider is found in Europe.

KEY ACTIONS

- ANTI-SPASMODIC
- EMOTIONALLY CALMING
- TREATS CYSTITIS
- PRESCRIBED FOR ANGINA

KEY PREPARATIONS

- TINCTURE made from the whole, live tarantula (or wolf) spider, macerated in alcohol and left to dissolve. The resulting solution is then succussed and diluted.

INDICATIONS

● **RESTLESS LIMBS**
Constant trembling and jerking of the hands and legs, usually random and unpredictable, such as that associated with multiple sclerosis, may be helped by this remedy. The spider and the remedy take their names from tarantism, a nervous disorder causing wild, uncontrollable body movements; the disease was popularly thought to be the result of being bitten by a wolf spider.

● **HEART CONDITIONS**
Tarentula treats angina and other heart disorders, where bodily trembling occurs, and sudden starts or thumping in the heart. Also prescribed for an irregular, infrequent pulse.

● **MOOD SWINGS**
Rapid mood changes, erratic behaviour, or sudden, violent, destructive actions can be calmed with this remedy.

● **WOMEN'S HEALTH**
Prescribed for sensitive genitalia with severe vulval itching, or where the vagina feels hot, dry, and raw.

● **CYSTITIS**
Treats the intense burning and stinging on urinating; controls a frequent urge to urinate, as well as possible incontinence when laughing or coughing.

ANTIMONIUM TART.

Heals skin conditions, including chicken pox

Treats exhaustion ◆ Alleviates nausea

Alchemists called this compound "tartar emetic" – it was traditionally prescribed as a powerful emetic.

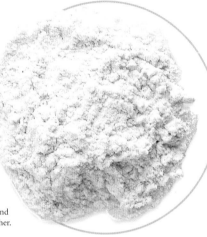

ANTIMONIUM POTASSIUM TARTRATE
This compound is commonly used as an insecticide and fix to bind dyes to textiles and leather.

ANTIMONIUM POTASSIUM TARTRATE POWDER AND LACTOSE SUGAR

KEY ACTIONS

- REDUCES EXHAUSTION
- PAIN-RELIEVING
- EASES BREATHING
- HEALS SKIN AILMENTS

KEY PREPARATIONS

- TINCTURE made by triturating antimony potassium tartrate with lactose sugar and then repeatedly diluting and succussing the mixture.

INDICATIONS

● **NAUSEA**
Known as the "prince of evacuants", this substance causes severe vomiting and was traditionally taken to expel intestinal worms. The remedy treats persistent nausea with trembling, weakness, and fainting.

● **HEADACHES**
Effective for headaches with pain that feels as if a tight band is constricting the head, possibly with weariness and a longing to close the eyes.

● **RESPIRATION**
Antimonium tart. is given for severe respiratory infection or chronic bronchitis. Also used to treat whooping cough.

● **CHICKEN POX**
Treats chicken pox and associated chest and digestive problems. Also heals the scars.

● **SKIN CONDITIONS**
Antimonium tart. is prescribed for acne and impetigo as well as chicken pox (*see above*). It is also used to treat warts.

● **EXHAUSTION**
Commonly given for strength-sapping illnesses in the young or elderly.

● **CAUTION**
Crystals of antimony potassium tartrate are poisonous.

THUJA

Alleviates urogenitary problems ◆ Treats catarrh
and sinusitis ◆ Heals painful skin conditions

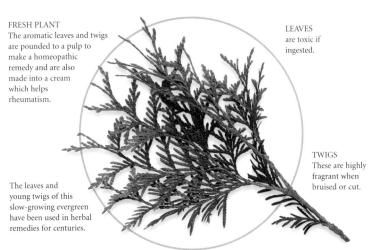

FRESH PLANT
The aromatic leaves and twigs
are pounded to a pulp to
make a homeopathic
remedy and are also
made into a cream
which helps
rheumatism.

LEAVES
are toxic if
ingested.

The leaves and
young twigs of this
slow-growing evergreen
have been used in herbal
remedies for centuries.

TWIGS
These are highly
fragrant when
bruised or cut.

KEY ACTIONS

- PAIN-RELIEVING
- ANTI-INFLAMMATORY
- HEALING

KEY PREPARATIONS

- SMOKE Native
  Americans burn
  Thuja (arbor vitae)
  for its smoky scent,
  which is deemed to
  ward off evil spirits.
- TINCTURE made from
  the fresh leaves and
  twigs of the one-
  year-old plant. They
  are chopped finely
  and macerated in
  alcohol, then
  filtered, diluted, and
  succussed.

INDICATIONS

● **HEADACHES**
Treats persistent neuralgic
pain due to exhaustion,
stress, or overexcitement,
or related to inflamed
gums, tooth decay, or
infected sinuses.

● **SKIN CONDITIONS**
Thuja is widely given for
warts and verrucas. Also
treats scaly, itchy skin
complaints and brown
"age spots". It is also
prescribed for ridged,
weak, or deformed nails.

● **MENSTRUATION**
Early or scant periods may
be treated with *Thuja*.
Also given for menstrual
pain that is localized in
the left ovary. Ovarian

cysts may also respond to
the remedy.

● **CATARRH & SINUSITIS**
Given for chronic sinus or
respiratory problems,
usually with catarrh.
Asthma may also respond
to *Thuja*.

● **URINARY PROBLEMS**
Relieves a swollen,
inflamed urethra, perhaps
with incontinence. Also
cures infection of the
urethra, possibly affecting
the prostate gland.

● **GENITAL DISORDERS**
Prescribed to clear up
genital discharges (in both
men and women), ulcers,
and uterine polyps. Also
treats genital warts,
gonorrhoea, and herpes.

GLONOINUM

Alleviates menopausal problems ◆ Promotes good
circulation ◆ Especially beneficial for the elderly

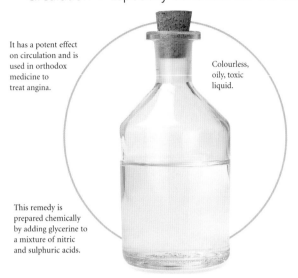

It has a potent effect
on circulation and is
used in orthodox
medicine to
treat angina.

Colourless,
oily, toxic
liquid.

This remedy is
prepared chemically
by adding glycerine to
a mixture of nitric
and sulphuric acids.

KEY ACTIONS

- REDUCES BLOOD
  PRESSURE
- CALMS HOT FLUSHES
- TREATS EXHAUSTION
- PRESCRIBED FOR
  HEADACHES

KEY PREPARATIONS

- TINCTURE made from
  nitroglycerine,
  dissolved in purified
  water, diluted, and
  succussed.

INDICATIONS

● **BLOOD PRESSURE**
Glonoinum, also known as
nitroglycerine, is
prescribed for patients
with high blood pressure.
It is used particularly to
treat the elderly.

● **CIRCULATION**
Symptoms that are treated
most effectively with
Glonoinum focus on the
regulation of the
circulation between the
head and the heart.

● **HOT FLUSHES**
This remedy is prescribed
when an increase in blood
supply causes flushes of
heat, similar to those
experienced during
heatstroke, which surge

up to the brain in waves,
resulting in severe
headaches (*see below*).
Glonoinum is also given
for hot flushes that occur
during menopause.

● **HEADACHES**
Homeopaths prescribe
Glonoinum for headaches
where there is typically a
bursting "full" sensation
in the head; this may be
accompanied by great
confusion and a
compulsion to hold the
head and squeeze it.

● **EXHAUSTION**
The remedy is prescribed
for heat exhaustion,
accompanied by a
throbbing, bursting
headache, sweaty skin,
and a hot face.

URTICA URENS

Soothes burning, painful skin conditions

Treats burns and scalds ◆ Given for nosebleeds

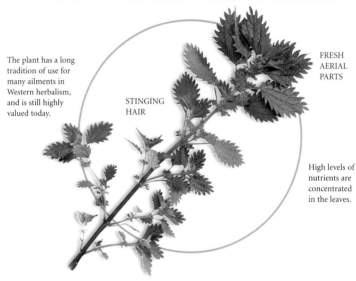

The plant has a long tradition of use for many ailments in Western herbalism, and is still highly valued today.

STINGING HAIR

FRESH AERIAL PARTS

High levels of nutrients are concentrated in the leaves.

KEY ACTIONS

- SOOTHING
- EASES PAINFUL MENSTRUATION
- ALLEVIATES ALLERGIES
- CALMS IRRITATED SKIN

KEY PREPARATIONS

- TINCTURE made from the whole flowering plant, including the root. It is steeped in alcohol.

INDICATIONS

● **URTICARIA**
Appropriately, urticaria – which is also known as nettle rash or hives – is a key condition treated by *Urtica urens*. The remedy relieves the red, burning, stinging skin eruptions that occur with the condition. The eruptions may be swollen or itchy and symptoms are often aggravated by warmth, bathing, or vigorous exercise. The itching tends to be worse on rising in the morning.

● **BLEEDING**
In the 1st century AD, the ancient Greek physician Dioscorides advocated this nettle and its relative,

Urtica dioica, as a treatment for nosebleeds and to help bring on delayed menstruation; it is also used to help heal festering wounds. The plant has a long tradition of use for many ailments in Western herbalism and is still valued highly by herbalists today.

● **SKIN CONDITIONS**
Given for blistering, burning, stinging, red, allergic rashes caused by insect bites, stings, eating shellfish, or contact with certain plants.

● **BURNS & SCALDS**
Urtica urens is given to treat burns or scalds accompanied by classic redness and blistering.

VERATRUM ALBUM

Treats symptoms of collapse ◆ Calms vomiting, nausea, and diarrhoea ◆ Used as a treatment for cholera

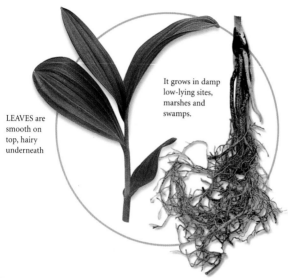

LEAVES are smooth on top, hairy underneath

It grows in damp low-lying sites, marshes and swamps.

ROOTSTOCK The fresh root is unearthed in autumn for use in homeopathic remedies.

KEY ACTIONS

- EASES CRAMP
- SAFE FOR USE IN PREGNANCY
- TREATS EMOTIONAL TRAUMAS
- HELPS DIGESTIVE DISORDERS

KEY PREPARATIONS

- TINCTURE made from the fresh root, dug up before flowering, chopped, macerated in alcohol, and succussed.

INDICATIONS

● DIARRHOEA

Along with *Camphor*, *Veratrum alb.* was successfully used to treat victims of the 19th-century cholera epidemic in Europe, helping to make Hahnemann's reputation. The remedy is used today to treat severe diarrhoea, possibly with vomiting or painful cramps, due to cholera, dysentery, gastroenteritis, or other digestive disorders.

● EMOTIONS

Prescribed for behavioural disorders, such as hyperactivity in children, adult insecurity, or emotional disturbances due to the trauma of childbirth.

● VOMITING & NAUSEA

Treats violent vomiting with nausea, clammy sweats and a cold feeling in the abdomen.

● COLLAPSE

For weakness with a clammy, sweaty forehead, blue-tinged skin, dehydration, and possible fainting. Can be used safely during pregnancy.

● CAUTION

The plant is toxic, although it is said that it is rare for fatality to occur from accidentally eating it as upon ingestion it instantly causes vomiting.

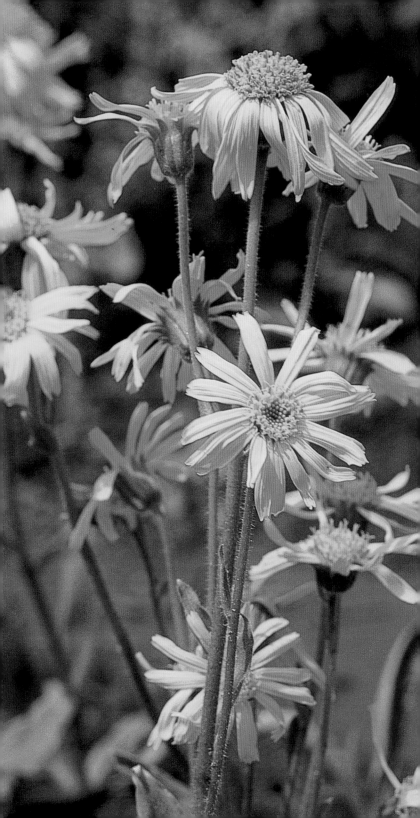

Homeopathic
Self-help

A self-help guide to determining the most

suitable homeopathic remedy for a range of

common complaints so that you can treat the

whole family through all stages of life.

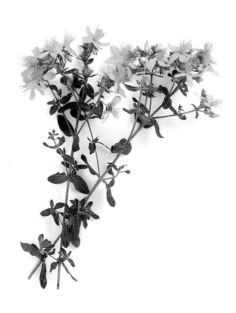

NERVOUS SYSTEM

With the use of homeopathy, the nervous system can be
gently healed, and recover its natural vitality.

DISORDER	AILMENT	SYMPTOMS
HEADACHE Headaches may indicate a serious ailment, but most are due to stress, fatigue, stimulants, allergy, eye strain, or low blood sugar. Pain results from strain on the head or neck muscles. **Self help:** For pain related to the neck, see a physiotherapist.	That comes on suddenly	• Pain may feel like a tight band • Head may feel full and heavy as though the brain is being pushed out • Possible pulsating or hot, bursting pain • Pain is possibly worse on the left side
	Caused by drinking too much alcohol	• Head feels as if it has been beaten • Dizziness, mental dullness, irritability • Bursting pain in the back of the head • Possible violent, jerking pain or dull, shooting pain in the left side of the brain
MIGRAINE A migraine usually occurs on one side of the head, and is associated with nausea, vomiting, blurred vision, or other visual disturbances such as zigzags, light intolerance, and sometimes tingling or numb arms. Symptoms are caused by the alternate constriction and swelling of the arteries supplying the brain. **Self help:** Avoid stress, learn relaxation techniques, and look into making dietary changes.	Worse on the right side of the head	• Pain in temples and the right side of the head; made worse by concentration • Possible dizziness, apprehension, anger • Lack of concentration • Memory appears to be failing
	Throbbing, blinding headache	• Preceded by numbness and tingling • Head feels stuffy, possibly with dizziness • Pain over eyes and on top of the head • Rejection of sympathy; desire to be alone • Tendency to dwell on sad memories
	With tearfulness	• Head feels as though it will burst • Pain starts in the right temple • Possible weeping of the right eye • Bruised sensation in the forehead • Tearfulness, timidity and desire for sympathy
SCIATICA This term describes pain that is transmitted along the sciatic nerve in the leg. It is caused by pressure on the nerve. **Self help:** Swimming may relieve the condition.	Worse in cold, damp weather	• Shooting pain down the right leg • Possible numbness, weakness, muscle contractions, and cramp-like pain • Irritability, anguish, or anger
	Relieved by heat and movement	• Tearing pain, numbness, and tingling • Pain extends down the back of the affected leg when passing stools • Cramp in the calf.

The nervous system is a huge and immensely complex structure, with the brain as the control centre. Nerve cells are vulnerable to damage, which can cause a range of problems from slight nerve twinges to stroke. Serious ailments require prompt conventional treatment, but there is a role for homeopathy's mind-and-body approach, especially during recuperation. The prescribed homeopathic remedies will treat the nervous system by calming the mind, thereby encouraging healing processes, as well as addressing specific symptoms.

SYMPTOMS BETTER	SYMPTOMS WORSE	REMEDY & DOSAGE
• In fresh air • For warmth • For rest • For perspiring	• In stuffy rooms • For colds and draughts • For a shock or fright • For light or noise	ACONITE (see page 31) 30c every 10–15 mins, up to 6 doses
• For warmth • For applying firm pressure • For washing the hair or applying cold compresses to the head	• In cold, dry, windy weather • Between 3 a.m. and 4 a.m. • For taking stimulants • For eating or physical or mental exertion	NUX VOMICA (see page 92) 6c every 10–15 mins up to 6 doses
• For loosening tight clothes • For movement • In cool air • For hot food and drinks • At night	• For wearing tight clothing • For overeating • In stuffy rooms • Between 4 a.m. and 8 a.m. and 4 p.m. and 8 p.m.	LYCOPODIUM (see page 77) 6c every 15 mins up to 10 doses after first signs
• In fresh air • For applying cold compresses to the head • For fasting • For lying down	• For warmth • For movement • In stuffy rooms • For grief	NAT. MUR. (see page 79) 6c every 15 mins up to 10 doses after first signs
• In cold, fresh, open air • For gentle movement • For crying	• For warmth • For rich or fatty foods • In the evening • During menstruation	PULSATILLA (see page 84) 6c every 15 mins up to 10 doses after first signs
• For applying firm pressure • For bending down • For heat • For rest or gentle movement	• In cold, wet weather • For emotional stress • Lying on the pain-free side • At night	COLOCYNTHIS (see page 55) 6c hourly up to 10 doses, or half-hourly if acute
• For heat • For continuous movement • For rubbing affected area • For stretching the limbs	• For rest • On moving for the first time after rest • For cold and damp	RHUS TOX. (see page 85) 6c hourly up to 10 doses, or half-hourly if acute

THE EYES

Homeopathic self-help remedies are particularly suitable for soothing tired, irritated, or infected eyes.

DISORDER	AILMENT	SYMPTOMS
EYE STRAIN Can be caused by overwork or working in poor light. Stress can also cause eye strain. **Self help:** Apply dry, cold compresses to the eyes or bathe them with Euphrasia solution (*see page 59*).	Eyes ache on movement	• Dull, aching pain in the eyes when looking up, down, or sideways • Aversion to sympathy or consolation • Possible symptoms associated with stress, especially after bereavement
	Burning eyes	• Eyes burn and feel strained after a prolonged period of studying or reading • Hot, red eyes; possible headache • Depression, anxiety, criticism of others
CONJUNCTIVITIS This results from infection (yellow discharge) or allergy (whites of the eyes are red and gritty). **Self help:** Bathe the eyes with Euphrasia solution (*see page 59*). Rest the eyes.	Swollen eyelids with burning discharge	• Eyes water continuously, which irritates skin below; eyelids swollen and burning • Frequent need to blink • Little blisters may form inside eyelids • Bland nasal discharge • Irritability
STYES A stye is a small, pus-filled boil at the base of an eyelash, caused by infection. It may be aggravated by tiredness. **Self help:** Rest the eyes and avoid touching them. Never squeeze a stye.	Inflamed eyes with itchy eyelids	• Eyes are red and swollen • Eyelids itch • Boils on the eyelids develop heads of pus • Depression, self-pity, possible tearfulness
	Inflamed and painful eyes	• Eyes are red, swollen, and painful • Boils on the eyelids develop heads of pus • Feelings of resentment or anger, especially concerning a loved one
WATERING EYES If constant, it may be caused by blocked tear ducts due to infection, or injury to the nose. **Self help:** Massage the sides of the nose.	Watering due to infection of tear duct	• Eyes water due to mild but persistent infection of the tear ducts • Lack of physical and mental stamina • Lack of confidence

The eyes are complex, delicate mechanisms. They are continually bombarded with atmospheric particles, such as spores, bacteria, viruses, chemicals and air pollutants, which may give rise to irritation and infection. Complaints in the eyes may be exacerbated by fluctuations in temperature, stress, and fatigue, all of which weaken the ability of the body's immune system to fight infection. Although homeopathic remedies will soothe eye problems, standard eye tests are essential for maintaining healthy eyes.

SYMPTOMS BETTER	SYMPTOMS WORSE	REMEDY & DOSAGE
• In fresh air • For fasting • For applying cold compresses	• In cold, thundery weather • In draughts or hot sun • For physical or mental exertion, or emotional stress	NAT. MUR. (see page 79) 6c 4 times daily up to 7 days
• For movement • For warmth • For gently massaging the eyes	• In cold, damp weather • For rest • When lying down • For drinking alcohol	RUTA (see page 86) 6c 4 times daily up to 7 days
• When the eyes are closed • For coffee	• In the evening • Indoors • For warmth • For light • In warm, windy weather	EUPHRASIA (see page 59) 6c hourly up to 10 doses
• For applying cold compresses to the affected area	• For rich, fatty foods • For hormonal changes, such as in puberty or pregnancy	PULSATILLA (see page 84) 6c hourly up to 10 doses
• For resting the eyes • For applying cold compresses to the affected area	• When the eye is touched • For the suppression of emotions, especially following a quarrel	STAPHYSAGRIA (see page 57) 6c hourly up to 10 doses
• For warmth • For applying warm compresses to the eyes • In summer	• In cold air and draughts • In damp conditions • For applying gentle pressure to the eyes • For mental exertion	SILICA (see page 88) 6c 4 times daily up to 7 days

THE EARS

Self-help remedies treat ailments linked to catarrh in the
ear, nose, and throat, resulting from respiratory infections.

DISORDER	AILMENT	SYMPTOMS
EARACHE This can result from a build-up of earwax or an infection – such as after a winter or summer cold. **Self help:** Hold a covered hot water bottle against the affected ear. **Caution:** If earache occurs with fever or discharge, see a doctor immediately. Consult a doctor about all earache in children.	With sharp pain	• Acute, throbbing pain • Extreme sensitivity to touch • Extreme irritability and anger • Emotional oversensitivity
	Throbbing earache with redness	• Bright red ear; throbbing pain • Wide, staring eyes • Restlessness and agitation, possibly with hallucinations or violent outbursts • High fever; dry mouth and throat
	Feeling of pressure behind eardrum	• Pain resulting from pressure behind the eardrum pushing it out slightly • Tearfulness and self-pity • Desire for company • In children, constant desire for cuddles
BLOCKAGE OF THE EUSTACHIAN TUBE This may become blocked by catarrh resulting from infection; by swollen adenoids; or after flying. **Self help:** Inhale three drops of lemon juice up each nostril three times daily for five days.	With coughing up of catarrh	• Deafness caused by swelling of the Eustachian tube • Cracking noise in the ear on blowing the nose or swallowing • Runny nose and coughing up of catarrh from the back of the throat • Irritability • Anger • Discontentment
TINNITUS Tinnitus is a persistent noise in the ears. It may be due to a foreign body in the ear canal, ageing, pressure damage, influenza, constant noise, stress, or taking certain drugs. **Self help:** Two drops of almond oil in each ear once a week.	Buzzing in the ears with dizziness	• Buzzing, especially in the left ear, sometimes accompanied by deafness and dizziness • Deafness accompanied by a severe headache and violent noise in the ears • Possible tenderness in the cervical or dorsal spine and pain in the head • Nervousness • Nominal aphasia (difficulty in naming objects) • Great anguish and fits of anxiety

The ears are intricate sensory organs that provide details to the brain about the body's external experiences, as well as controlling balance. An ear has an outer, a middle, and an inner section, which relay and interpret sound waves. The ears are susceptible to invasion by particles and micro-organisms and are easily damaged, so any pain or other kind of discomfort should be investigated promptly. Homeopathic remedies can be of particular help in treating ailments linked to catarrh resulting from respiratory infections.

SYMPTOMS BETTER	SYMPTOMS WORSE	REMEDY & DOSAGE
• For warmth • For applying warm compresses to the head • When the head is warm	• In cold air and draughts • When the ear is touched • When lying on the affected side	**HEPAR SULPH.** (see page 65) 6c half-hourly until you see a doctor
• When standing or sitting upright • For applying cold compresses to the forehead	• When the head is chilled • For movement, jarring, noise, light, or pressure • When lying on the right side	**BELLADONNA** (see page 40) 30c half-hourly until you see a doctor
• For gentle movement • In fresh air • In cool, dry conditions	• In hot, stuffy conditions • In the evening • When lying on the left side • For prolonged reading	**PULSATILLA** (see page 84) 6c hourly up to 10 doses
• For cold drinks • For gently rubbing the ear	• In fresh air • In draughts • When lying down at night • In damp conditions	**KALI. MUR.** (see page 72) 6c 4 times daily up to 7 days
• For applying pressure to the ear • For yawning • When bending forwards	• At precise, regular intervals • For cold • Between 10 a.m. and 11 a.m. • For touch • For movement	**CHINA** (see page 52) 6c 3 times daily up to 14 days

RESPIRATORY SYSTEM

By building a strong immune system, homeopathic remedies help the body to ward off respiratory infections.

DISORDER	AILMENT	SYMPTOMS
HAY FEVER AND ALLERGIC RHINITIS Hay fever may be caused by seasonal irritants such as grass, tree, and flower pollens. Allergic rhinitis refers to those symptoms that occur year round. **Self help:** Avoid all known irritants.	With burning catarrh	• Catarrh may begin in the left nostril • Pain in the forehead • Possible pain in the larynx • Eyes stream, causing irritability
	In which the eyes are mainly affected	• Swollen, light-sensitive eyes • Burning discharge that irritates the skin beneath, causing mental irritability • Bland catarrh that drips down the back of the throat
COUGH & COLDS Colds are caused viral infections. They are usually self-limiting, but may worsen if neglected. A cough is the body's attempt to expel an irritant from the respiratory tract. **Self help:** Rest and drink plenty of fluids. Eat plenty of fresh vegetables and fruit. Get some fresh air. **Caution:** If there is pain or breathing difficulties, consult a doctor.	Colds that come on slowly	• Mouth feels hot; throat is inflamed • Mild fever; excitability • Nose may bleed
	A cold with irritablity	• Chilliness; headache; sore throat • Nose is runny by day, blocked by night • Watering eyes and sneezing
	Early stages of a cough or cold	• Violent sneezing and thin catarrh • Possible blocked nose or cold sores • Desire to be alone; aversion to sympathy
	Irritating cough that comes on suddenly	• Dry, hollow-sounding, croaky cough • Great thirst • Possible rapid rise in temperature • Extreme anxiety
INFLUENZA The influenza virus has many strains. The whole body is usually affected. **Self help:** Rest and drink frequently. Eat fresh fruit and vegetables. **Caution:** If fever persists for four days, see a doctor.	With weakness	• Chills running up and down the spine • Shakiness and trembling; anxiety • Bursting headache, relieved by urinating • Fever; brain feels drowsy; fatigue
	With a high fever	• Fever comes on suddenly • Flushed face; wide, staring eyes • Confusion, delirium, horrible visions • Bright red, sore throat

With every breath we take, spores, viruses, bacteria, and microscopic particles of dust, smoke, and chemical pollutants enter the body. The respiratory system is therefore highly susceptible to the effects of atmospheric irritants. Colds, coughs, and influenza strike easily when the immune system is weak, making the body vulnerable. The immune system may be impaired by exposure to cold or windy weather or weakened by overwork, exhaustion, anxiety, and stress. Homeopathy helps to keep the body's natural defences intact.

SYMPTOMS BETTER	SYMPTOMS WORSE	REMEDY & DOSAGE
• In cool rooms or fresh air • For bathing • For movement	• In warm rooms • In cold or damp weather • For warm foods and drinks	**ALLIUM CEPA** (see page 33) 6c as required up to 10 doses
• When lying down in a darkened room • For coffee	• For warmth • In warm, windy weather • For bright light • Indoors • In the evening	**EUPHRASIA** (see page 59) 6c as required up to 10 doses
• For cooling the forehead • For gentle exercise • For lying down	• For jarring and touch • In fresh air and sun • Between 4 a.m. and 6 a.m.	**FERRUM PHOS.** (see page 61) 6c 2 hourly up to 4 doses
• For warmth and sleep • In the evening • For firm pressure to nose	• In dry, cold wind • For emotional stress • For spicy food or stimulants	**NUX VOMICA** (see page 92) 6c 2 hourly up to 4 doses
• In fresh air • For fasting • For cooling the sinuses	• In cold, thundery weather • For mental exertion • In draughts, sea air, or sun	**NAT. MUR.** (see page 79) 6c 2 hourly up to 4 doses
• In fresh air • For movement • For warmth	• Exposure to smoke or pollen • In the evening and at night • In cold, hot, or windy weather	**ACONITE** (see page 31) 30c every 4 hours up to 10 doses
• In fresh air • For urinating • For applying hot compresses to head and neck	• In the sun • In humid conditions • For emotional stress	**GELSEMIUM** (see page 62) 6c every 2 hours up to 10 doses
• When standing or sitting upright • In warm rooms	• For jarring and movement • For noise, light, and heat • At night • Lying on the right side	**BELLADONNA** (see page 40) 30c every 2 hours up to 10 doses

CIRCULATORY SYSTEM

Problems caused by poor circulation benefit from a complete health programme that includes homeopathy.

DISORDER	AILMENT	SYMPTOMS
CHILBLAINS Chilblains occur when superficial blood vessels contract excessively because of cold. **Self help:** Keep hands and feet as warm and dry as possible. Apply calendula ointment. Do not scratch. Take regular exercise.	Burning, itchy chilblains	• Skin in affected areas is red, prickly, and swollen • Intolerable itching and burning pain • Great anxiety about health
	Chilblains with swollen veins	• Burning, throbbing pain in affected areas and bluish inflammation • Biting, itching sensation if scratched • Possible tearfulness due to discomfort
CRAMP Cramp is acute pain that occurs when muscles go into spasm. It may occur after prolonged sitting, standing, or lying awkwardly. **Self help:** Stretch the muscles and massage them to increase the blood supply.	Severe cramp in the legs or feet	• Muscle twitching leading to violent muscle spasms • Ankles are painfully heavy • Knees bend involuntarily when walking • Tearfulness and anxiety
	Cramp from muscle fatigue	• Pain resembling bruising • Limbs are heavy and feel as though they have been beaten • Fear of being touched • Oversensitivity to noise
VARICOSE VEINS Varicose veins occur when the veins start to fail and pools of blood build up. They may be hereditary, or result from obesity, pregnancy, or thrombosis. **Self help:** Stand as little as possible and wear support tights. Sit with the feet raised above the hips. **Caution:** If it persists for three weeks, see a doctor.	With a sore, bruised feeling	• Veins are inflamed, possibly with burning feeling, and feel bruised and tender to the touch • Veins may bleed and are sore, swollen, and lumpy • Irritability and anxiety
	Worse for sitting with legs hanging down	• Veins feel full • Chilliness • Veins smart and sting • Timidity and submissiveness • Tearfulness with desire for reassurance

CIRCULATORY SYSTEM

The circulatory system transports blood around the body, supplying body tissues with oxygen and nutrients. As well as homeopathic self-help remedies for specific ailments, homeopathic treatment according to constitutional type may improve the body's general metabolic function, reduce stress, and maintain the health of other organs. Circulatory disorders benefit most from a complete health programme that includes homeopathic treatment as well as a healthy diet, exercise, and a lifestyle that avoids smoking and overwork.

SYMPTOMS BETTER	SYMPTOMS WORSE	REMEDY & DOSAGE
• For slow movement • When warm in bed	• On exposure to cold and damp • In cold weather • Before thunderstorms	**AGARICUS** (see page 32) 6c half-hourly up to 6 doses
• With the hands above the head • For gentle exercise • In cold, fresh air	• For heat • In extremes of temperature • In the evening and at night	**PULSATILLA** (see page 84) 6c half-hourly up to 6 doses
• For applying firm pressure to the affected area • For cold drinks • For perspiring	• For movement • For applying light pressure to the affected area • During sexual intercourse	**CUPRUM MET.** (see page 56) 6c 4 times daily up to 14 days
• On starting to move • In clear, cold weather • When lying down	• For heat • For applying light pressure to the affected area • For prolonged movement	**ARNICA** (see page 39) 6c 4 times daily up to 14 days
• For rest • For lying down quietly • In winter	• For injury • For movement or jarring • For applying pressure to the affected area • In warm, humid weather	**HAMAMELIS** (see page 64) 30c twice daily up to 7 days
• In cold, fresh air • For applying cold compresses • When standing upright • When lying on the back	• For warmth • In the evening • During pregnancy	**PULSATILLA** (see page 84) 30c twice daily up to 7 days

THE MOUTH

Most problems can be prevented by good oral hygeine and diet, but minor disorders respond well to self-help remedies.

DISORDER	AILMENT	SYMPTOMS
TOOTHACHE Often an indication of tooth decay, but it may also be a symptom of infection, such as gum disease or an abscess. **Self help:** Rub oil of cloves on to the affected tooth and gums, except when taking another homeopathic remedy.	With severe, shooting pain	• Oversensitivity to pain • Jerking, tearing pain that makes sleeping difficult
	With unbearable pain	• Agonizing pain; swollen, red cheeks • Irritability; irascibility
	With throbbing pain	• Gums and cheeks are swollen and painful to the touch • Shoooting pains extending to the ears • Waves of pain that increase in severity
GINGIVITIS The gums bleed and become darker, swollen, and infected. Usually due to poor brushing, but may also be due to stress or other medical conditions. **Caution:** If there is no improvement after three days, see a doctor.	Bleeding gums with halitosis	• Gums are tender, spongy, and bleed easily; teeth may feel loose • Excessive production of saliva • Mental dullness; lack of motivation • Hesitant speech; slow comprehension
	Swollen, bleeding gums with ulcers	• Taste of pus in the mouth • Teeth are very sensitive to heat and cold • Possible mouth ulcers or cold sores • Aversion to sympathy; desire to be alone
HALITOSIS Halitosis, or bad breath, can be caused by tooth decay, smoking, gingivitis, indigestion, tonsillitis, sinusitis, or fasting. **Self help:** Avoid food with a strong odour.	Associated with tooth decay and gingivitis	• Breath and sweat smell offensive • Excessive productionof saliva • Tongue is yellow and thickly coated • Aversion to sympathy; desire to be alone
MOUTH ULCERS These are inflamed spots inside the mouth. **Self help:** Avoid spicy, sweet, or acidic foods. **Caution:** If ulcers have not healed in three weeks, seek medicinal help.	Burning mouth ulcers	• Mouth feels dry • Smarting, burning soreness in ulcerated areas • Metallic or bitter taste in the mouth • Tongue is clean, dry, and red • Restlessness and anxiety

THE MOUTH

Problems with teeth and gums are common in developed countries, where the diet is rich in sugar. Many mouth problems can be prevented by regular dental check-ups. good oral hygiene, and a diet that includes fibrous, chewy, non-sugary foods that help to stimulate the production of saliva, which contains infection-fighting white blood cells. Homeopathic treatment for oral infections include soothing mouthwashes for conditions such as gingivitis and mouth ulcers as well as standard remedies that depend on specfic symptoms.

SYMPTOMS BETTER	SYMPTOMS WORSE	REMEDY & DOSAGE
• For ice-cold water in the mouth • For lying down	• For heat • For hot foods • For noise	COFFEA (see page 53) 6c 4 times daily for 14 days
• For sympathy • For cooling the area	• At night • For being angry	CHAMOMILLA (see page 50) 6c 4 times daily for 14 days
• For rest • For leaning the head against something • For bending backwards	• For touch • For jarring • At night • In fresh air	BELLADONNA (see page 40) 30c every 5 mins up to 10 doses
• For rest • When warmly dressed • In the morning	• In extremes of temperature • For perspiring at night • For stress • In draughts	MERC. SOL. (see page 66) 6c every 4 hours up to 3 days
• In fresh air • For fasting • For rubbing the affected area	• For physical or mental exertion, or emotional stress • For warmth and in hot sun	NAT. MUR. (see page 79) 6c every 4 hours up to 3 days
• For rest • When warmly dressed • For rubbing the gums	• For cold and extremes of temperature • For perspiring at night • For stress	MERC. SOL. (see page 66) 6c 3 times daily up to 7 days
• For a warm mouthwash • For applying warm compresses to the face • When lying with the head higher than the body	• For cold foods and drinks • In cold, dry, windy weather • Between midnight and 2 a.m. • For stress • For being run down	ARSEN. ALB. (see page 28) 6c 4 times daily up to 5 days

DIGESTIVE SYSTEM

Minor ailments, such as indigestion lend themselves to self-help, especially if combined with dietary controls.

DISORDER	AILMENT	SYMPTOMS
INDIGESTION Indigestion is a blanket term for a number of symptoms, including burping, stomach ache, and heartburn. **Self help:** Practise some form of relaxation or meditation before you eat. Do not rush your food and relax after eating.	With excessive flatulence	• Digestion seems to have slowed down • Pain when eating even the plainest food • Burning feeling in the stomach
	With painful retching	• Craving for fatty, acidic, or spicy foods and alcohol, which upset the digestion • Heartburn 30 minutes after eating
	With nausea and/or vomiting	• Possible headache around the eyes and feeling of pressure under the breastbone • Tearfulness, depression, and self-pity
HEARTBURN Heartburn is a common form of indigestion consisting of a burning pain in the stomach or oesophagus and the chest. **Self help:** Try relaxation or meditation before you eat. Eat calmly and relax for 30 minutes afterwards. Avoid eating late and avoid foods that you know upset you. If you smoke, stop.	With desire for ice-cold water	• Burning sensation in the chest • Craving for ice-cold water • Constant hunger
	With craving for sweets	• Laziness and lack of mental energy • Burning sensation from hunger.
	Vomiting and diarrhoea together	• Vomiting with burning pain in the abdomen • Diarrhoea that causes soreness of the anus and stinging in the rectum • Craving for cool drinks that may be vomited up
GASTROENTERITIS This inflammation of the digestive tract is caused by a virus in contaminated food or water. **Self help:** Rest and drink plenty of fluids (salted, cooled, boiled water). Avoid drinking milk or eating any solid food until the stomach settles. **Caution:** If symptoms persist, see a doctor.	With severe abdominal cramps	• Colicky pains that are better when the body is bent double • Pain relieved by passing wind • Possible diarrhoea

DIGESTIVE SYSTEM

A healthy, efficient digestive system is essential for both physical and mental well-being, but it can be upset by many factors. Some can be controlled, such as diet and, to a certain extent, emotional stress or allergy, and some cannot, like inherited problems. Homepathic remedies are concerned with improving the condition of the digestive tract, by adjusting the number of beneficial bacteria; reducing irritation caused by some foods; improving waste elimination; and maintaining the organs involved in the digestive process.

SYMPTOMS BETTER	SYMPTOMS WORSE	REMEDY & DOSAGE
• For burping • In cold, fresh air	• For overeating • For rich, fatty foods • For eating too late	**CARBO VEG.** (see page 47) 30c every 10–15 mins up to 7 doses
• For warmth • For sleep • For being alone	• For touch • For fatty, acidic, or spicy foods or alcohol	**NUX VOMICA** (see page 92) 6c every 10–15 mins up to 7 doses
• For gentle exercise • For crying	• For rich, fatty foods • For emotional stress • In hot stuffy conditions	**PULSATILLA** (see page 84) 6c every 10–15 mins up to 7 doses
• For cold foods and water • For sleep • For general body massage	• When lying on the back • For stress • For warm foods	**PHOSPHORUS** (see page 82) 6c every 10–15 mins up to 7 doses
• In the open air • For warm drinks	• For bathing • When standing up	**SULPHUR** (see page 93) 6c every 10–15 mins up to 7 doses
• For hot drinks • For warmth	• At the sight and smell of food • Between midnight and 2 a.m. • For cold drinks • For alcohol	**ARSEN. ALB.** (see page 28) 6c hourly up to 10 doses
• When lying on one side with the knees pulled up to the chest • For warmth and sleep	• For eating or drinking • In cold, damp weather • At around 4 p.m.	**COLOCYNTHIS** (see page 55) 6c hourly up to 10 doses

SKIN DISORDERS

Homeopathic practitioners look for the underlying causes of skin problems and the factors that aggravate the skin.

DISORDER	AILMENT	SYMPTOMS
MILD ACNE This includes blackheads, whiteheads, and yellowheads. It may be caused by stress, certain drugs, or hormones. **Self help:** Sunlight in moderation and fresh air.	Painful, pus-filled spots	• Yellowheads which are extremely painful to the touch • Irritability and petulance
	Associated with hormonal imbalance	• Spots occur during puberty • Tearfulness and self-pity • Associated with delayed or scanty menstruation in adolescent girls
MILD ECZEMA This is common, especially in children. It may be exacerbated by stress, hormonal changes, or dietary factors. **Self help:** Avoid known irritants. Wear cotton next to the skin.	With restlessness	• Skin is dry and burning, but is aggravated by cold compresses • Restlessness and inability to sit still • Sleeplessness, especially after midnight • Possible anxiety and need for reassurance
	Dry eczema	• Skin is rough, red, and itchy • Possible diarrhoea • Craving salty, fatty, spicy, or sweet foods • Anxiety and lack of mental energy
BOILS A boil is a firm swelling (nodule) beneath the skin caused by infection of a hair follicle. They may be associated with illness, being run-down, fatigue, or stress. **Self help:** Clean the skin. Never squeeze a boil. Avoid handling food after dealing with boils.	Early stages of formation	• Possible sudden onset of symptoms • Boil is hard and round • Skin around the boil is dry, inflamed, painful, and throbbing • Possible fever, inducing delirium
	Later stages, when pus has formed	• Boil has a head of pus that is on the point of bursting • Boil is sensitive to the slightest touch • Possible extreme bad temper • Desire for no physical or emotional contact
COLD SORES Cold sores are caused by a virus and triggered by being run-down or by hot, cold, or windy weather. **Self help:** Avoid eating peanuts, chocolate, seeds, and cereals.	On the lips and around the mouth	• Mouth feels dry • Lips are swollen and burning, with pearl-like blisters • Blisters weep before becoming crusty • As blisters dry up they may develop into deep, painful cracks • Depression; aversion to sympathy; desire to be left alone

SKIN DISORDERS

The skin accounts for 60 per cent of the total body. Homeopathic practitioners tend to regard skin complaints as an outer manifestation of what is going on within the body, and look for underlying causes of skin eruptions. Stress, poor diet, hormonal imbalance, and allergies, as well as infections may all cause outbreaks. Skin conditions may be aggravated by factors such as lack of exercise; eating sugary foods, refined carbohydrates, or other foods; caffeine and alcohol; constipation; the use of cosmetics; and contact irritants in the environment.

SYMPTOMS BETTER	SYMPTOMS WORSE	REMEDY & DOSAGE
• For heat • In damp weather • For eating	• When the spots are touched, even lightly • For cold	HEPAR SULP. (see page 65) 6c 3 times daily up to 14 days
• For crying • In the open air • For applying cold compresses	• For rich, fatty foods • In warm, stuffy rooms • For hormonal changes	PULSATILLA (see page 84) 6c 3 times daily up to 14 days
• For warmth • For applying warm compresses • For walking around	• For cold • Between 12 a.m. and 2 a.m. • For physical or mental exertion • For drinking milk	ARSEN. ALB. (see page 28) 6c 4 times daily up to 7 days
• In fresh air • For cold • For perspiring	• For washing • For becoming overheated • Early in the morning	SULPHUR (see page 93) 6c 4 times daily up to 7 days
• For applying pressure to the affected area • At night • For warmth	• For applying cold compresses • In draughts • For touch	BELLADONNA (see page 40) 30c hourly up to 10 doses
• For warmth • For applying warm compresses to the affected area • In damp weather	• In cold air and draughts • For even the lightest touch • When lying on the affected area	HEPAR SULPH. (see page 65) 6c hourly up to 10 doses
• In fresh air • For fasting	• At around 10 a.m. • In cold, thundery weather • For warmth, hot sun, sea air, or draughts • For noise, music, or talking • For jarring • For physical or mental exertion	NAT. MUR. (see page 79) 6c 4 times daily up to 5 days

EMOTIONAL HEALTH

Homeopathic treatments are used to help stimulate a
person's natural ability to cope with emotional problems.

DISORDER	AILMENT	SYMPTOMS
INSOMNIA Insomnia describes a persistent pattern of intermittent sleep that leaves the sufferer feeling tired and unrefreshed.	With inability to relax	• Sudden onset of insomnia • Overactive mind • Sleep occurs eventually but is fitful • Possible painful headache
Insomnia can be caused by being unwell, sleeping in an airless environment, excess of caffeine or alcohol, overexcitement,	With irritability	• Wakefulness between 3 a.m. and 4 a.m. then more settled sleep just before it is time to get up; possible nightmares • Craving for stimulants • Constipation with ineffectual urging
stress, food allergy, shock, or anxiety. **Self help:** Increase your amount of exercise. Avoid	With great fear	• Nervousness; restlessness; nightmares • Sudden onset of insomnia • Fitful sleep caused by pain • Numbness in the limbs
eating late in the evening. Stop work an hour before bedtime and relax. **Caution:** If there is no improvement within three weeks, consult a doctor.	With fear of never sleeping again	• Continuous yawning but unable to sleep • Lump in the throat • Growing apprehension about going to bed; possible nightmares • Rapid changes of mood
IRRITABILITY & ANGER These emotions are often a response to events that are perceived to be physically or psychologically threatening. They can be	Irritability with over- critical attitude	• Anger that comes on quickly • Awkwardness and intractability • Sensitivity to the cold • Desire for alcohol and fatty or spicy foods • Overcriticism of others
brought on by overwork, overindulgence, digestive ailments, exhaustion, or impotence in men. They may lead to depression. **Self help:** Increase your amount of exercise. Practise relaxation techniques.	Anger with insecurity	• Craving for sweet foods • Feeling of hunger but full up after a few bites • Lack of self-confidence

Homeopathy, on its own, is well suited to the treatment of emotional problems. As a holistic form of medicine it examines all aspects of the individual – physical, intellectual, spiritual – and a practitioner does not separate these elements when prescribing treatment. Homeopathic treatment for emotional problems helps people cope in the short term but, in the long term, it is best combined with dietary changes, regular exercise, relaxation techniques or movement therapies, and stress management in order to maximize the benefits of the treatment.

SYMPTOMS BETTER	SYMPTOMS WORSE	REMEDY & DOSAGE
• For warmth • When lying down • For sucking ice	• For taking sleeping pills • For strong smells • For noise • In fresh air or the cold	COFFEA (see page 53) 30c hourly before bed for 10 nights
• When lying on either side • When sitting • For warmth • In the evening	• When lying on the back • For overeating, especially spicy foods • In cold, windy weather • For noise	NUX VOMICA (see page 92) 30c hourly before bed for 10 nights
• In fresh air • For warm perspiration	• In warm rooms • On exposure to tobacco smoke • For loud music	ACONITE (see page 31) 30c hourly before bed for 10 nights
• For eating • For urinating • For walking around	• In fresh air • For cold • For coffee and alcohol	IGNATIA (see page 69) 30c hourly before bed for 10 nights
• For warmth • For sleep • In the evening	• For cold • For noise • For overeating • At around 4 a.m.	NUX VOMICA (see page 92) 6c half-hourly up to 10 doses
• For sleep • For cool conditions • For hot foods and drinks • After midnight	• In stuffy rooms • For wearing tight clothing • For overeating • Between 4 p.m. and 8 p.m.	LYCOPODIUM (see page 77) 6c half-hourly up to 10 doses

CHILDREN'S HEALTH

Remedies are easily administered to babies and children
and can help them bounce back to health quickly.

DISORDER	AILMENT	SYMPTOMS
COLIC Believed to be a painful spasm of the intestines. **Self help:** If breast-feeding, avoid certain foods.	With crying relieved by warmth	• Bloated abdomen • Distress, restlessness, and irritability • Sudden onset of gripping or shooting pains in the stomach • Pains not relieved by burping
NAPPY RASH The skin may become red and sore due to contact with soiled nappies. **Self help:** Wash the baby's skin with a solution of calendula and hypericum.	Dry rash on sensitive skin	• Skin is dry, red, scaly, and irritated • Desire to scratch as soon as a nappy is removed
	Intensely itchy rash with blisters	• Redness and blisters • Restlessness and a desire to scratch as soon as a nappy is removed
TEMPER TANTRUMS Caused by emotional stress, teething, or allergies. **Self help:** Discipline a child consistently.	Child is impossible to please	• Cheeks may be red if the child is teething; irritability • Possible convulsive symptoms • Oversensitivity to pain • Dislike of being talked to or touched
GLANDULAR FEVER This is spread by personal contact. Symptoms subside in two to three weeks, but full recovery may take longer. **Self help:** Rest in bed till acute symptoms abate. **Caution:** See a doctor to confirm diagnosis.	With offensive perspiration	• Throat is dark red, sore, and swollen • Irritability and emotionalism • Saliva burns the throat on swallowing • Tongue is yellow-coated and feels swollen • Bad-smelling breath and perspiration
	With pain on swallowing food and hot drinks	• Tonsils are dark red • Shooting pain up to the ears on swallowing • Restlessness and indifference
BODY ODOUR Sweat glands become functional in adolescence. The odour becomes offensive when bacteria breed in the sweat. **Self help:** Wash every day using alkaline soap.	In overweight people who feel the cold	• Perspiration smells sour • Profuse perspiration overnight and in the morning, and for moderate exertion • Depression, apprehension, and anxiety
	Perspiring in hot and cold conditions	• Copious, unpleasant-smelling perspiration that occurs in hot and cold conditions

Childhood extends from one to twelve years old. During this period the immune system prepares itself for puberty and adulthood. Parents often prefer to treat their children with gentle, natural products to reduce the risk of side effects, resorting to conventional drugs only when a child's immune system is unable to cope with a serious ailment.

Following on from childhood, many of the common disorders found in adolescents result from hormonal changes. Homeopathic remedies can help address these bodily imbalances.

SYMPTOMS BETTER	SYMPTOMS WORSE	REMEDY & DOSAGE
• For warmth • For warm baths • For applying light pressure to the stomach	• In cold air • At night • For touch • When lying on the right side	MAG. PHOS. (see page 78) 6c every 5 mins up to 10 doses
• In fresh air • When warm and dry	• For wearing too much clothing or being too warm • For being washed	SULPHUR (see page 93) 6c 4 times daily up to 5 days
• For changing position • When warm and dry	• For being undressed • For getting wet • In draughts	RHUS TOX. (see page 85) 6c 4 times daily up to 5 days
• For being carried • For perspiring • In mild weather	• When teething • At night • After breakfast • For being talked to	CHAMOMILLA (see page 50) 30c daily up to 7 days
• For rest • When warmly dressed • In the morning	• In extremes of temperature • For perspiring • At night • When lying on the right side	MERC. SOL. (see page 66) 6c every 4 hours up to 10 doses
• For rest • When lying on the stomach • For warmth	• For getting out of bed • For movement • For swallowing • For hot foods and drinks	PHYTOLACCA (see page 83) 6c every 4 hours up to 10 doses
• In dry weather • In the morning • After breakfast	• For cold • For mainly physical but also mental exertion	CALC. CARB. (see page 44) 6c hourly up to 10 doses
• For rest • In the morning	• In extremes of temperature • For perspiring • At night	MERC. SOL. (see page 66) 6c hourly up to 10 doses

ADULT HEALTH

Both men and women with problems relating to the
reproductive cycle, respond well to homeopathic treatment.

DISORDER	AILMENT	SYMPTOMS
PREMENSTRUAL SYNDROME (PMS) PMS affects about 75 per cent of women and includes psychological and physical symptoms. Self help: Avoid salty, fatty, or junk foods, sugar, tea, coffee, and alcohol. Take daily exercise.	With apathy, irritability, and tearfulness	• Greasy skin, possibly with acne • Craving for salty or sweet foods • Weariness, fits of anger, and screaming • Reduction in sex drive • Sensation as though uterus is falling out
	With swollen, tender breasts	• Fluid retention • Swollen, tender breasts and painful joints • Lack of energy; depression; indifference • Possible vaginal discharge or thrush
PAINFUL PERIODS Also known as Dysmenorrhoea. Discomfort is common during the first few days of a period. Self help: Eat plenty of raw fruits and vegetables. Take plenty of exercise. Lose weight if necessary.	Abdominal pain with depression and self-pity	• Cramp in the uterus causing nausea or vomiting; tenderness in the abdomen • Depression; migraine. desire for comfort • Tearing pain in the abdomen
	Abdominal pain soothed by heat and pressure	• Colicky, spasmodic pain • Irritability, anxiety, fixation about pain • Blood flow includes clots • Dark, stringy, and tarry blood flow • Period starts ahead of schedule
ERECTILE DYSFUNCTION Problems with erection may result from physical causes, or from stress. Self help: Try to relax. Caution: If symptoms persist, see a doctor.	In anticipation of failure	• Penis remains cold and small • Possible premature ejaculation • High sex drive, but lack of self-confidence
	Caused by bruising	• Penis is bruised after an injury • Penis feels sore and tender to the touch • Possible premature ejaculation • Fear of being touched
BALINITIS The medical term for swelling and soreness of the foreskin and glans penis, possibly caused by friction or irritation. Self help: Keep clean. Use calendula ointment.	With inflamed foreskin and glans penis (head of the penis)	• Inner surface of the foreskin is irritated and inflamed • Possible itching • Possible ulceration • Possible discharge of offensive-smelling pus

There is much anecdotal evidence of homeopathy's success in treating women's complaints. Homeopathic remedies can provide an attractive alternative to conventional treatments such as hormone replacement therapy (HRT) – and are particularly suitable for the treatment of recurring ailments associated with the reproductive cycle. For men, many conditions are easily treated if diagnosed early, and respond well to homeopathy. Neglect, on the other hand, can lead to complications that threaten fertility, sexual function, and even life.

SYMPTOMS BETTER	SYMPTOMS WORSE	REMEDY & DOSAGE
• For eating • For sleep • For vigorous exercise • For heat	• For cold • For tobacco smoke • For mental exertion • In the early morning and early evening	**SEPIA** (see page 87) 30c twice daily up to 3 days, from 1 day before PMS due
• In the morning • When slightly constipated	• In draughts • In cold, damp, and wind • For overexertion • Between 2 a.m. and 3 a.m.	**CALC. CARB.** (see page 44) 30c twice daily up to 3 days, from 1 day before PMS due
• For crying and sympathy • For gentle exercise • In fresh air • For cold drinks	• For heat • In extremes of temperature • For rich, fatty foods • In the evening and at night	**PULSATILLA** (see page 84) 30c hourly up to 10 doses
• For warmth • For hot baths • For applying pressure to the abdomen • When bending double	• In cold air and draughts • For being uncovered • At night • For being exhausted • For movement	**MAG. PHOS.** (see page 78) 30c hourly up to 10 doses
• For loosening clothing • For warm drinks • For urinating	• For wearing tight clothing • In very hot rooms • For overeating	**LYCOPODIUM** (see page 77) 30c twice daily up to 5 days
• For bathing in cold water • For adopting a sexual position that avoids pressure on the bruised area	• For touch • For further injury or bruising • For sexual excesses	**ARNICA** (see page 39) 30c twice daily up to 5 days
• In moderate temperatures • For rest • For scratching the affected area • In the morning	• At night • For perspiring • For overheating • In cold air and draughts	**MERC. SOL.** (see page 66) 6c every 4 hours up to 5 days

INDEX

CKNOWLEDGMENTS

PUBLISHER'S ACKNOWLEDGMENTS
Dorling Kindersley would like to thank Franziska Marking for picture research, Hilary Bird for compiling the index, and Marshall Baron for proof reading.

PHOTOGRAPHY
The publisher would like to thank the following for their kind permission to reproduce their photographs:

a=above; c=centre; b=below; l=left; r=right; t=top
AKG London: 13; Erich Lessing 10, 12.
Geoscience Features: Dr. B. Booth 82.
Magnum: Hiroji Kubota 24bl.
N.H.P.A.: Jany Sauvanet 9, 74.
Science Photo Library: CNRI 18c.
Superstock Ltd.: 25br.
Telegraph Colour Library: Paul Aresu 19b; Ancil Nance 25tr;
Adam Smith Production 18b; Stephen Simpson 19t.

All other photography by Steve Gorton, Neil Fletcher, Matthew Ward, Andy Crawford, Harry Taylor, Phillip Dowel, Colin Keates, Dave King, Martin Cameron, Anne Hyde, Jonathan Buckley, Deni Bown, Howard Rice, David Murray, Roger Phillips, and Peter Chadwick.